Question Bank on Veterinary Public Health and Food Safety

The Author

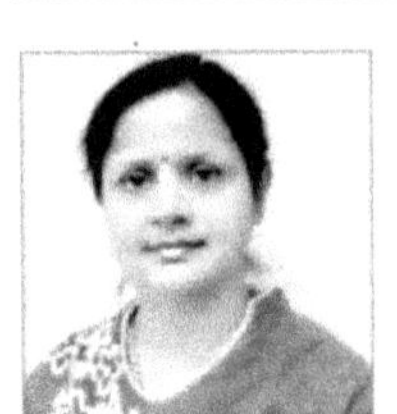

Dr. Namita Joshi, is Professor and Head, Department of Veterinary Public Health and Epidemiology at College of Veterinary Science and Animal Husbandry, Narendra Deva University of Agriculture and Technology, Faizabad (UP). Dr. Joshi graduated in 1992 in Veterinary Science and Animal Husbandry from G.B. Pant University of Agriculture and Technology, Pantnagar (Uttrakhand). She did her Master's degree and Ph.D. from the same university in year 1994 and 2001, respectively. Dr. Joshi has been associated with teaching of Veterinary Public Health and Epidemiology in G.B. Pant University of Agriculture and Technology, Pantnagar and N.D. University of Agriculture and Technology, Faizabad for last 10 years. She has about 50 research papers to her credit published in reputed National and International Journals and developed two manuals for under graduate students on 'Milk and Meat Hygiene, Food Safety and Public Health' and 'Veterinary Epidemiology and Zoonoses'. Dr. Joshi has been elected member of Indian Association of Veterinary Public Health Specialists. She is also Assistant Editor in the Journal of Immunology and Immunopathology and acting as reviewer in many journals.

Question Bank on Veterinary Public Health and Food Safety

for Ready Reference to the Students, Teachers and Researchers, Civil Service Examinations (State and Central), NET, Ph.D. and Allied Examinations

Namita Joshi

Daya Publishing House®
A Division of
Astral International Pvt. Ltd.
New Delhi – 110 002

Cataloging in Publication Data—DK
Courtesy: D.K. Agencies (P) Ltd. <docinfo@dkagencies.com>

Joshi, Namita *(Professor of veterinary public health and epidemiology)*, **author.**
Question bank on veterinary public health and food safety : for ready reference to the students, teachers and researchers, civil service examinations (state and central), NET, Ph.D. and allied examinations / Namita Joshi.
pages cm
ISBN *9789351246565 (Int. Edition)*

1. Veterinary public health—India—Examinations, questions, etc. 2. Food—India—Safety measures—Examinations, questions, etc. 3. Veterinary hygiene—India—Examinations, questions, etc. I. Title.

SF740.J67 2017 DDC 636.0832 23

Published by : **Daya Publishing House®**
A Division of
Astral International Pvt. Ltd.
– ISO 9001:2008 Certified Company –
4760-61/23, Ansari Road, Darya Ganj
New Delhi-110 002
Ph. 011-43549197, 23278134
E-mail: info@astralint.com
Website: www.astralint.com

प्रो. अख़्तर हसीब
कुलपति
Prof. Akhtar Haseeb
Vice-Chancellor

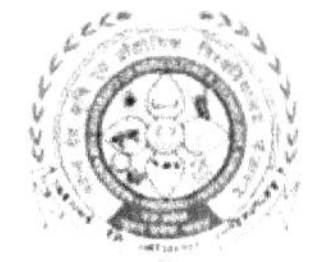

नरेन्द्र देव कृषि एवं प्रौद्योगिक विश्वविद्यालय
कुमारगंज, फैजाबाद - 224 229 (उ.प्र.)
भारत
Narendra Deva University of Agriculture & Technology
Kumarganj, Faizabad-224 229 (U.P.) INDIA

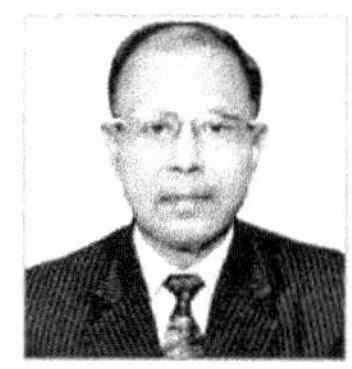

Foreword

Veterinary public health is a multidisciplinary subject that caters needs of all aspects of health. All the issues pertaining to animal, human and environmental health are well addressed within the ambit of veterinary public health. Veterinary Public Health directly improves human health by reducing exposure to hazards arising from interactions with animals and animal products. Examples of these hazards include zoonoses, vector-borne infections and other communicable diseases, chemicals and veterinary drugs used in animals, envenomations, and injuries from occupational and recreational exposure to animals. Although the concept of Veterinary Public Health originated in 1940 at Centre for Disease Control and Prevention, Atlanta, USA. Later, it was recognized as essential component of public health activity in 1975 by the expert committee of FAO/WHO. Since then, the scope of Veterinary Public Health has been expanding all over the world. Keeping pace with rapidly growing and changing world, Veterinary Council of India, the statutory body of Government of India, has introduced Public Health in Veterinary course curriculum and created a separate department of Veterinary Public Health. The VCI has implemented Minimum Standard of Veterinary Education-Degree course (B.V.Sc. & A.H.) Regulation, 1984, to regulate the veterinary undergraduate education. Thus, the subject of veterinary public health became an imperative part of veterinary education. Since, the Department of Veterinary Public Health came in existence in many colleges in late 1990s only after the implementation of VCI Regulations; both teachers and students face difficulties in procuring the study material of the subject.

The objective of an enhanced VPH curriculum is to provide graduates of all learning backgrounds with up-to-date knowledge and expertise, so that they can actively contribute to VPH programmes. Dr. Namita Joshi, Professor and Head, Department of Veterinary Public Health and Epidemiology has very timely identified the difficulties; the students are facing in competitive examinations and created this question bank with their answers to provide readymade supplementary material for competitive examination. The book comprises 4 chapters on Veterinary Public Health and Food Hygiene, Milk Hygiene, Meat Hygiene and Environmental Hygiene covering almost all aspects of Veterinary Public Health. The questions are coined very meticulously and ready answers are provided at the end of each chapter.

I am confident that her efforts in the form of book entitled "Question bank on veterinary public health and food safety" will prove very useful for the veterinary graduates and teachers. I wish that all veterinary students make full use of this compilation for their own benefit and the benefit of the society as a whole.

(Akhtar Haseeb)

Preface

Veterinary Science has helped in reducing animal suffering, minimizing risk of zoonotic diseases threatening human health and food security. There have been unprecedented advancement in the branches of veterinary science in fast few decades. The futuristic requirement of society on public health, food safety and quality, healthy ecosystem, containing bioterrosism, profitability and stability of livestock farming system have posed greater challenges to veterinary academician and scientific community. Today, veterinarian are increasingly involved in prevention and control of zoonoses and emerging pathogens, eco-health stewardship, monitoring and surveillance of animal diseases, combating bioterrorism, genetic engineering to optimize production, develop disease resistant breeds of animals and handle the vetero-legal cases of speciation. All these issues pertaining to animal, human and environmental health are well addressed within the ambit of veterinary public health. Because veterinary public health is a multidisciplinary subject that encompasses knowledge of food hygiene, ecology, environmental hygiene, zoonoses and epidemiology, pathbiology, molecular biology besides public health education and administration. In a broader sense, it covers every aspect of veterinary activities related to human health. In this perspective, significant modifications have been made in the syllabus of under graduate courses by Veterinary Council of India and post-graduate courses by Indian Council of Agricultural Research to respond to futuristic social need. Although, at undergraduate level, veterinary students acquire comprehensive knowledge and skills in all veterinary courses but the students aspiring for higher education, JRF and/or ARS/NET examination need a consolidated question bank of veterinary public health courses. This book in a way is an outcome of long term study and teaching in veterinary public health at undergraduate and post-graduate levels. The book will provide opportunity to the students to prepare themselves as per the need of hour and to understand their lacunae in the field of public health. The contents of the book have been organized into four chapters *viz.* Food Safety and Veterinary Public Health, Food Hygiene, Milk Hygiene, Meat Hygiene and Environmental Hygiene. I hope the students and teachers in the field of veterinary public health would find the organization of book useful and encourage the student to do more exhaustive study.

I take this opportunity to express my gratitude to Dr. Akhtar Haseeb, Vice Chancellor of Nrandera Dev University of Agriculture and Technology, Kumarganj for his constant inspiration and encouragement to veterinary faculty. I also thank Dr. H.N. Singh, Dean, College of Veterinary Science & A.H. for his kind support.

At last, I am very much grateful to my husband Dr. R.K. Joshi for giving his time to time valuable suggestions. My vocabulary utterly fails in expressing my accolade to my mother Smt. Kamla Pant, who brought me upto this stage. I am also grateful to my kids Trishala and Pushpit for their cooperation and forbearance.

Namita Joshi

Contents

Chapter 1

Veterinary Public Health and Food Hygiene

MULTIPLE CHOICE QUETIONS

1. **The most ancient Indian text in which rules and regulations for public health, dietetics and hygienic ritual at the time of birth and death, have been prescribed is:**

   (a) Charak Samhitas (b) Harit Samhitas

   (c) Susruta Samhitas (d) Manu Samhitas

2. **Hygeia was regarded as the Goddess of :**

   (a) Health (b) Cleanliness

   (c) Hygiene (d) All of above

3. **Public health is an art and science of _______ through organized community efforts.**

   (a) Preventing disease (b) Prolonging life

   (c) Promoting Health (d) All of above

4. **The concept of happiness has its roots in ancient Indian philosophy and the comprehensive concept of health is found in:**

   (a) Atharveda (b) Ayurveda

   (c) Samveda (d) Yajurveda

5. **Concept of 'one medicine' was proposed by:**
   (a) Martin Kaplan (b) Calvin W. Schwabe
   (c) John Snow (d) Willium Furr

6. **The Veterinarian whose contribution facilitated the development of modern public health policies in the domain of food hygiene is:**
   (a) Bernhard Bang (b) Edward Jenner
   (c) Daniel Salmon (d) Jacob Nufer

7. **The 'National Institute of Communicable Diseases' (NICD) is situated at_______:**
   (a) Banglore (b) New Delhi
   (c) Bhopal (d) Kolkata

8. **The 'National Institute of Communicable Diseases' (NICD) has been renamed as_______:**
   (a) National Centre for Disease Control
   (b) National Communicable Disease Centre
   (c) National Infectious Disease Research Centre
   (d) National Centre for Public Health

9. **Which one of the following is not a member of public health unit at district level in India?**
   (a) Chief Veterinary Officer (b) Chief Medical Officer
   (c) Teacher (d) Revenue Collector

10. **Which one of the following is not a member of public health unit at block level in India?**
    (a) Physician (b) Veterinarian
    (c) Sanitary Engineer (d) Revenue Collector

11. **The health services in India are organized at three levels. District hospitals are _______ service provider.**
    (a) Primary health care (b) Secondary health care
    (c) Tertiary health care (d) None of above

12. Community development programme of Panchyati Raj was launched with the aim to exterminate the.

(a) Poverty (b) Disease

(c) Illiteracy (d) All of above

13. All the developmental programmes of Panchayati Raj in villages are channelized through

(a) Gram Panchayat (b) Panchayat samiti

(c) Jila Parishad (d) All of above

14. The common epidemiological approach for Veterinarian and public health practitioner to disease management is

(a) Prevention (b) Control

(c) Treatment (d) Eradication

15. The following are common features of Veterinary and public health practices to disease management except one

(a) Population concept (b) Economic consideration

(c) Disease prevention (d) Disease Eradication

16. OIE was established in the year:

(a) 1924 (b) 1954

(c) 1934 (d) 1964

17. The chief of OIE is called as:

(a) Chairperson (c) Director General

(b) President (d) Chief Executive Officer

18. The Head Office of OIE is situated at:

(a) Paris (b) Rome

(c) Geneva (d) Manila

19. Dr. Bernard Vallet is presently working as Director General of _______ from 2000.

(a) WHO (b) FAO

(c) WTO (d) OIE

20. The general sessions of OIE are held annually in the month of_______.

(a) January (b) May

(c) June (d) September

21. The organizational governance of OIE is mediated by three main bodies. The one which is not concerned with this, is:

(a) Administrative commission

(b) Regional commission

(c) Specialist commission

(d) Codex Alimenterius Commission

22. The VPH section of WHO is principally concerned with

(a) Zoonoses (b) Comparative medicine

(c) Food Hygiene (d) All of above

23. The Head Quarter of Regional Centre of WHO for Southeast Asia is situated at

(a) Islamabad (b) New Delhi

(c) Beijing (d) Bangkok

24. According to joint FAO/WHO expert committee, the principle public health function of Veterinarian is/are

(a) Animal related (b) Journalist

(c) Biomedical (d) All of above

25. Headquarter of WTO is situated at _______, Switzerland.

(a) Paris (b) Rome

(c) Geneva (d) Manila

26. The agreements of WTO that facilitate the international trade and resolve trade dispute related to livestock product is:

(a) AOA (b) TBT

(c) SPS (d) All of above

27. WTO member countries must establish official contact points for communicating about SPS measures. These contact points are known as:

(a) National enquiry point

(b) National Notification authority

(c) Both of above (d) None of above

28. The Quarantine Act was promulgated in India in the year:

(a) 1825 (b) 1850

(c) 1857 (d) 1947

29. The presence of the animal disease that imposes trade embargo in India is:

(a) Foot and Mouth Disease (b) Haemorrhagic Septicemia

(c) Black Quarter (d) Haemorrhagic Colitis

30. SPS measures provide protection not only from introduction and spread of diseases but also from______ in foods.

(a) Pests (b) Toxins and contaminants

(c) food additives (d) All of above

31. The structural framework of WTO is very extensive but highest decision making body is.

(a) Ministerial conference

(b) General council

(c) Secretariat

(d) Committees of specific issues

32. WTO acts as forum for the governments ______:

(a) To negotiate trade agreement (c) To operate trade rules

(b) To settle trade dispute (d) All of above

33. 'Codex Alimenterius Commission' was established in the year_______.

(a) 1960 (b) 1962

(c) 1964 (d) 1970

34. 'International Organisation for Standardisation' promotes world-wide _______ standard.

(a) Proprietary (b) Industrial

(c) Commercial (d) All of above

35. 'International Organisation for Standardisation' has formulated standards for food in relation to:

(a) Food hygiene (b) Food microbiology

(c) Food quality assurance (d) All of above

36. ISO 14000 family addresses _______ standard.

(a) Environment management

(b) Quality management

(c) Information security management

(d) Risk Management

37. ISO 27000 family addresses _______ standard.

(a) Environment management

(b) Quality management

(c) Information security management

(d) Risk Management

38. BIS is a founder member of:

(a) WHO (b) FAO

(c) WTO (d) ISO

39. The Head Quarter of BIS is situated at:

(a) Chandigarh (b) New Delhi

(c) Kolkata (d) Chennai

40. Food protection activity of Veterinarian are related towards prevention of:

(a) Animal diseases

(b) Residues in food of animal origin

(c) Chemicals in food of animal origin

(d) All of above

41. Which one is most important among the following major issues pertaining to food safety?

(a) Microbiological hazards

(b) Chemical hazards

(c) Surveillance of food borne diseases

(d) New technologies

42. Most of the potential food hazards can be controlled along the food chain through

(a) Good agricultural practices

(b) Good manufacturing practices

(c) Good hygienic practices

(d) All of above

43. Which one is most important and difficult for developing country to address food safety?

(a) Microbiological and chemical hazard

(b) Capacity building

(c) Surveillance of food borne diseases

(d) New technologies

44. Which of the following cause of food safety problems is considered to be an unconventional agent?

(a) Naturally occurring toxins

(b) Persistent organic pollutants

(c) Bovine spongiform encephalopathy

(d) Heavy metals

45. Following are the key principle in strengthening national food control systems but one of them is the foundation on which food control policies are based.

(a) Integrated farm to table concept

(b) Regulatory Impact assessment

(c) Transparency

(d) Risk analysis

46. Risk analysis at international level is carried out by

(a) JECFA (b) JMPR

(c) JEMRA (d) All of above

47. Microbiological Risk analysis comprises three components; which one is not part of it.

(a) Risk assessment (b) Risk characterization

(c) Risk communication (d) Risk management.

48. Which step is not part of risk assessment process?

(a) Hazard identification (b) Risk characterization

(c) Hazard characterization (d) Risk management.

49. Food Safety and Standard Regulation was operationalised on 5th August______.

(a) 2010 (b) 2006

(c) 2011 (d) 2008

50. All the following are critical features of Food safety and standard act which were not included in PFA act in decision making except one.

(a) Stakeholder involvement (b) Multiple authorities

(c) Risk assessment (d) Science based standards

51. The objective of Food safety and standard authority of India is to regulate ______ of food products.

(a) Manufacture (b) Sale and import

(c) Storage and distribution (d) All of above

52. The factor that must be considered for devising attribute sampling scheme is/are.

(a) Microbiological incidence (b) Type of hazard

(c) Processing technique (d) All of above

53. A criterion incorporated in a regulation, controlling food production, processing or storage or import into the area of jurisdiction is called:

(a) Microbiological Criterion (b) Microbiological Limit

(c) Microbiological Standard (d) Microbiological Specification

54. A criterion recommended by an authority for adoption in a specific region but not incorporated into law is called:

(a) Microbiological Criterion

(b) Microbiological Limit

(c) Microbiological Standard

(d) Microbiological Specification

55. A microbiological values established by use of defined procedures and applied in acceptance of sampling of food is called:

(a) Microbiological Criterion

(b) Microbiological Limit

(c) Microbiological Standard

(d) Microbiological Specification

56. Three class sampling plan is applied to those organisms that pose:

(a) No direct health hazard

(b) Low indirect health hazard

(c) Moderate direct hazard

(d) All of above

57. In three class sampling plan, the value that denotes maximum safety limit and separates marginally acceptable quality from defective quality is:

(a) M

(b) N

(c) m

(d) C

58. All the following pathogens have been placed in the category of severe hazard as per ICMSF except:

(a) *Salmonella typhi*

(b) *Salmonella typhimurium*

(c) *Salmonella paratyphi*

(d) *Shiegella dysenteriae*

59. All the following pathogens have been placed in the category of severe hazard as per ICMSF except:

(a) *Clostridium botulinum*

(b) *Vibrio cholerae*

(c) *Brucella melitensis*

(d) *Staphylococcus aureus*

60. *Trichenella* has been placed in which category of microbiological hazard as per ICMSF:

(a) Severe (b) Moderate

(c) Low (d) None of above

61. *Coxiella burnetti* has been placed in which category of microbiological hazard as per ICMSF:

(a) Severe (b) Moderate

(c) Low (d) None of above

62. Which of the following microbial toxicity is associated with the aquatic food?

(a) *Vibrio parahaemolyticus* (b) Scarlet fever

(c) Botulism (d) *Staphylococcus aureus*

63. The food born intoxication that takes place due to unhygienic handling is caused by:

(a) *E. coli* (b) *Salmonella*

(c) *Campylobacter* (d) *Staphylococcus aureus*

64. Minamata disease is caused by ingestion of fish contaminated with:

(a) Mercury (b) Lead

(c) Cadmium (d) Arsenic

65. The effects of cyanide on thyroid and nervous system are observed in the person as a consequence of long term consumption of inadequately processed:

(a) Potato (b) Seafood

(c) Milk (d) Cassava

66. APEDA is mandated with the responsibility of export promotion of:

(a) Poultry and poultry product (b) Meat and meat product

(c) Dairy product (d) All of above

67. The concept of HACCP was for the first time introduced by:

(a) H.E. Bauman (b) James Jay

(c) Edwards and Ewing (d) Charles Badwin

68. HACCP approach exercises control measures towards prevention of any _______ of microorganism in production chain.

(a) Objectionable contamination (b) Survival

(c) Multiplication (d) All of above

69. The major critical control point in processing of milk and milk products is:

(a) Bactofugation (b) Pasteurization

(c) Homogenization (d) Cooling

70. The time elapsed between preparation of first dilution and pouring of medium in the last plate in SPC method should not be more than.

(a) 10 minutes (b) 30 minutes

(c) 20 minutes (d) 40 minutes

71. In drop method, _______ drops of standard volume of the dilutions are transferred to the dry surface of solid agar medium from a height of 2.5 cm.

(a) Two (b) Four

(c) Six (d) Eight

72. In spread plate count method, _______of various dilutions is taken as inoculums.

(a) 0.1 ml (b) 0.2 ml

(c) 1.0 ml (d) 0.01 ml

73. In drop method, inoculum is transferred to the surface from a height of_______.

(a) 0.5 cm (b) 1.5 cm

(c) 2.5 cm (d) 3.5 cm

74. If the plates are showing no colonies of bacteria in1:100 dilution, the result should be interpreted as:

(a) Zero/ml (b) Less than one/ml

(c) Less than 100/ml (d) 100/ml

75. Which of the following medium exhibits pink colonies of *Salmonella* surrounded by red medium?

(a) Bismuth sulphite agar (b) Heketoen enteric agar

(c) Brilliant green agar (d) Salmonella Shiegella agar

76. Which of the following test is more appropriate to detect pathogenic *Staphylococci*?

(a) Coagulase (b) Haemolysis

(c) Phosphatase (d) Thermonuclease.

77. Which of the following shows synergistic effects in CAMP test with *Staphylococcus aureus?*

(a) Listeria monocytogenes (b) Listeria welshimeri

(c) Listeria ivanovii (d) *Listeria innocua*

78. Which of the following is not used as enrichment medium for Salmonella?

(a) Tetrathionate broth (b) Buffered peptone water

(c) Rappaort-Vassiliadis (d) Selenite broth

79. The generation time of the microorganisms will be shortest during:

(a) Lag phase (b) Stationary phase

(c) Log phase (d) Decline phase

80. Thermal death point is the lowest temperature at which all microbes in suspension will be killed in _______:

(a) 10 minutes (b) 15 minutes

(c) 20 minutes (d) 30 minutes

81. The time of heating at a temperature to cause 90 per cent reduction in the count of viable cells or spores is called:

(a) D value (b) Z value

(c) F value (d) None of the above

82. The canning industry has recommended 12D concept of heat treatment for _______ spores in low acid food as a safety measure.

(a) Cl. perfringen (b) *Cl. botulinum*

(c) Cl. noyii (d) *Bacillus cereus*

83. The commercial refrigeration temperature *i.e.* lower than 5°C, effectively retard the growth of many food borne pathogens except:

(a) *Clostridium botulinum* type E

(b) Clostridium botulinum type A

(c) *Bacillus cereus*

(d) *Clostridium perfringens*

84. The temperature at which botulism toxin is destroyed in 10 minute is:

(a) 30°C (b) 80°C

(c) 100°C (d) 121°C

85. Antibiotics are mostly used as preservative in ______ food to lengthen the storage time at chilling temperature:

(a) Carbohydrate (b) Proteinecious

(c) Fatty (d) All of above

86. Halogens/Hypochlorites are used for the treatment of water used for______ in plant:

(a) Drinking purpose (b) Processing purpose

(c) Washing purpose (d) All of above

87. The concentration of chlorine used for sanitization purpose in food plant should be:

(a) 0.5 to10 ppm (b) 10 to 20 ppm

(c) 20 to100 ppm (d) 100 to 200 ppm

88. The concentration of chlorine in processing water of food plant should be:

(a) 0 to 0.5 ppm (b) 0.5 to 10ppm

(c) 10 to 20 ppm (d) 20 to100 ppm

89. The disinfection action of chlorine is mainly due to:

(a) Hypochlorite (b) Hypochloric acid.

(c) Hypochlorous acid (d) None of above

90. The concentration of chlorine in water used for sanitizing purpose in food processing plant should be :

(a) 0.5 to 10 ppm (b) 0 to 0.2 ppm

(c) 10 to 20 ppm (d) 100 to 250 ppm

91. Sugar and salts exert microbicidal effect by:

(a) Reducing water activity

(b) Ionizing to yield chloride ion

(c) Increasing osmotic pressure

(d) All of above

92. Wood smoke contains large number of volatile compounds that may have bacteriostatic and bactericidal effect but most effective one is :

(a) Formaldehyde (b) Cresol

(c) Phenol (d) Aliphatic acid

93. Which of the following irradiation process is equivalent to thermal processing of canned food?

(a) Radurization (b) Radicidation

(c) Radappertiztion (d) Hurdle technology

94. The factor(s) that influences the effectiveness of UV rays is/are:

(a) Time (b) Penetrability

(c) Intensity (d) All of above

95. The intensity of light in food plant at inspection side should not be less than:

(a) 550 LUX (b) 110 LUX

(c) 220 LUX (d) 50 LUX

96. The Cleaning and sanitization procedure of equipments surface is said to be satisfactory if colony count/900 sq.cm area is :

(a) < 5000 (b) > 25000

(c) 5000 to 25000 (d) None of above

97. Bacteria and virus that cause serious diseases in humans but for which vaccines or other treatment exist are placed in the category of

(a) Biohazard level 1 (b) Biohazard level 2

(c) Biohazard level 3 (d) Biohazard level 4

98. The agents whose characteristics are not fully understood or poorly understood are placed in the category of

(a) Biohazard level 1 (b) Biohazard level 2

(c) Biohazard level 3 (d) Biohazard level 4

99. Which one of the following is not related to biohazard level 2:

(a) Hepatitis virus (b) Variolla virus

(c) Influenza A virus (d) Salmonella

100. N_{95} respirator is required in biosafety level:

(a) One (b) Two

(c) Three (d) All of above

FILL IN THE BLANKS

1. The word hygiene is derived from Greek word Hygeia which means_______.
2. Hygeia was the daughter of the god of medicine named as _______.
3. Word 'Sanitation' is derived from a Latin word _______ meaning _______.
4. The most ancient Indian civilization showing the relics of practices of environmental sanitation is_______.
5. The cities of Indus valley civilization that showed the evidence of drainage, bath and sewerage system in excavation are_______ and_______.
6. Concept of 'one medicine' denotes intimate relationship between_______ and_______.
7. Unit of concern in public health is_______.
8. The first Veterinary school was established at_______ in 1762 by Claude Bourglat.
9. The concept of Veterinary public health was evolved at _______ in 1942.

10. Veterinary Public Health was recognized as an important component of public health by FAO/WHO in ______.
11. Veterinary Public Health is defined as sum of all contributions to ______, ______ and ______ of human through application and understanding of Veterinary knowledge.
12. A Veterinary public health practitioner relies on ______ to diagnose the disease.
13. The first international standard setting body that was granted general consultative status with UN economic and social council and also concerned with food safety is known as ______.
14. ISO was established in 1946 after union of two organizations, ______ and ______.
15. The abbreviation 'ISO' for 'International Organisation for Standardisation' is derived from Greek word ______ meaning equal.
16. ISO 9000 family addresses ______ standard.
17. The international organization that is mainly concerned with the health of consumers and formulation of various specifications for hygienic food production is ______.
18. The name of US agency that implements regulations related to animal products safety is ______.
19. USDA has assigned the responsibility of animal product safety regulation to ______.
20. The organization that assists international community in development of guiding principle for animal welfare is ______.
21. 'Office International des Epizootics' is also known as ______.
22. The first Director General of OIE was ______ from 1927-1949.
23. The joint Food Standard Program of FAO and WHO resulted in the establishment of ______ to protect the health of consumer.
24. The main objective of CAC is to develop ______ standards.
25. The main objective of OIE is to develop ______ standards.

26. There are _______ regional commissions, _______ specialist commissions and _______ administrative commission in OIE.
27. Activities of OIE are supported by _______ commission and number of working groups made up of international experts.
28. Out of four specialist commission of OIE, three work close together to deal with animal diseases while one commission deals with _______.
29. The Director General of OIE and members of OIE commissions are appointed by _______.
30. The various resolutions of OIE are passed by _______ at annual general session.
31. Rapid exchange of animal disease information between the countries is mediated by _______.
32. Three sister organizations which develop international standards that are valid under SPS agreement are _______, _______, _______.
33. The first school of public health in Southeast Asian region was established in Kolkata in 1932 with the name _______
34. The national institute that is responsible for surveillance and monitoring of animal diseases in India is _______.
35. PD-ADMAS has been renamed as 'National Institute of _______'.
36. The 'High security animal disease laboratory' has been renamed as _______.
37. Rural areas in India have been organised into blocks that comprise approximately_______ villages.
38. A block usually comprises of about _______ population.
39. The urban areas of a district are organized into three types of administrative institution *viz.* _______, _______, _______.
40. Three tier structure of local governance in India that links villages to districts is _______.
41. The Panchayati Raj agency at village level is called the _______.
42. The Panchayati Raj agency that works at block level is called _______.

43. The Panchayati Raj agency that works at district level is called _______.

44. The most important health programme of Govt. of India launched in 2005 to provide effective health care to rural people was _______.

45. The international organization that deals with global trade rules is known as _______.

46. World Trade Organization was established in 1995 as a successor to _______ (agreement).

47. WTO member countries must establish official contact points to enhance _______.

48. Providing appropriate technical assistance and education tools for food safety initiatives is called _______.

49. The concept of risk assessment was first introduced in _______ agreement of WTO in1995.

50. Codex standards, guidelines and recommendations are explicitly recognized under _______ agreement and qualify as "international standard" under_______ agreement of WTO.

51. Food safety was recognized as essential public health function in _______ world health assembly in _______ to develop global strategy.

52. Food safety programmes are increasingly focussing on the _______ approach.

53. Most scientific and systematic approach used in risk assessment is _______.

54. Correction of hazards at various stages of production and processing is termed as _______.

55. Adulteration of milk in India is an offence and it was previously punishable under _______ Act.

56. The authority established with the aim of laying down the science based standards for article of foods in India is _______.

57. Consumer empowerment is a salient feature of _______ Act, under which consumers can take samples of food and get it analyzed.

58. Microbiological specifications for meat and meat products, milk and milk products, poultry, seafood and eggs have been suggested by _______.
59. As per ICMSF, the criterion 'M' denotes_______ for number of bacteria that is considered safe in food.
60. In ICMSF, value 'm' denotes _______ for number of bacteria in sample units.
61. The attribute sampling schemes comprise two main things; _______ and _______.
62. 'Two class sampling plan' denotes two attributes, *i.e.* _______or _______ of organism in a given sample unit.
63. 'Three class sampling plan' has three attributes, *i.e.*_______, _______ and _______.
64. _______ sampling plan is applied to more hazardous type of organism.
65. _______ sampling plan is applied to moderately or less hazardous type of organism.
66. The pathogens that pose moderate direct hazard and have extensive spread potential are subjected to _______ sampling plan.
67. C is the number of sample units where bacterial count may be between_______.
68. The value of C in two class sampling plan is usually _______.
69. The value of C in three class sampling plan ranges between _______.
70. Group of organisms that indicate likely presence of a hazard in food and water but they, themselves may or may not be responsible for the hazard are called _______.
71. The food samples should be transported as rapidly as possible within _______.
72. The refrigerated food samples should not be stored for more than _______ (time) for microbiological testing.
73. The light intensity in food safety laboratory should not be less than_______.

74. For bacteriological examination, temperature of molten agar media should be brought down to _______ for plating.

75. Medium used for selective isolation of *Cl. perfringen* in food and water is _______.

76. _______ agar medium is used for the detection of Coliforms in a food sample.

77. The test performed to determine the commercial sterility of processed canned food is _______.

78. Black colonies of *Salmonella* surrounded by narrow green margin are seen on _______ medium.

79. 'Anton's test' is performed to test the pathogenecity of _______.

80. Medium which is used for selective isolation of *E. coli* O157:H7 is called as _______.

81. 'Kanagawa reaction is performed on _______ media to test the virulent *Vibrio parahaemolyticus*.

82. The isolates identified as *Vibrio cholerae* should be submitted for serotyping to _______ (lab).

83. The ability to prevent deposition of undesirable mineral salts on surfaces being cleaned is called_______.

84. The carcinogenic substance that is formed in food as a result of nitrite treatment is _______.

85. The destruction of food enzymes by heat is called _______.

86. The strength of the sewage in food plant waste is expressed in terms of _______.

87. _______ detergents are widely used to remove milk stone and water scales.

88. _______ has excellent deflocculating and emulsifying properties.

89. A British scientist, who developed 'tyndallization' process for germ reduction in food, was _______.

90. _______ and _______ are primarily used as sterilants for packaging material and fumigation of warehouse.

91. Sterilization doses or heavy doses of radiation cause _______in pH of meat.

92. Meat, poultry and fish can be perfectly sterilized with _______ kilogray dose of radiation so that they can be kept at room temperature for long time.

93. A term used to label foods treated with low level ionizing radiations is _______.

94. Microbial metabolite that is used as indicator of quality of fish is _______.

95. Organo-chlorine pesticides (OCL) are not readily excreted by animal body due to their _______ nature.

96. The extra amount of chlorine from water is removed by adding _______.

97. The poisoning which is thought to be caused by ingestion of fish having histamine as result of bacterial degradation is called _______.

98. The temperature of the water for sanitizing the dairy equipments should be_______.

99. _______beyond the break point may be employed to areas or equipments where slime bacteria may be a problem.

100. _______is a term used in microbial thermal death time calculations. It is the temperature required for one log10 reduction in the D-value.

MARK TRUE/FALSE

1. As per WHO, health is defined as a state of complete physical, mental and social well being of living thing.

2. The principle unit of administration in India is the district.

3. Head of municipal board is called Mayor while head of corporation is called Chairman.

4. Panchayati Raj is a three 3 tier structure of rural local self governance in India linking villages to the state.

5. In India, Panchayati Raj institutions are accepted as public welfare agencies ensuring more effective participation of the people in governance.
6. The block is considered as basic unit of rural planning and development in the state.
7. All community development programmes (CDP) are executed by Jila Paishad, however Panchayat Samiti is simply a supervisory body.
8. The head of Panchayat Samiti is called as Community Development Officer.
9. All the funds released by government for stage I and stage II development in villages are channelled through Panchayat Samiti.
10. Community development programme was launched in1952 for all round development of the urban areas.
11. The programme launched after CDP to eliminate rural poverty and improve the quality of life was known as 'Integrated rural development programme (IRDP)'.
12. The 'Integrated rural development programme' (IRDP) was proposed to provide self employment opportunities to rural people through district rural development agency.
13. Most of the states in India do not have independent Veterinary public health units.
14. District Animal Husbandry officer is a team member of public health unit at block level.
15. Veterinary public health services in India started with the establishment of 'Division of Zoonoses' at IVRI in 1964.
16. First caesarian section on a woman was performed successfully by a veterinarian named Jacob Nufer.
17. The epidemiological approach of a veterinary practitioner and a public heath practitioner for disease investigation is more or less similar and that is host oriented rather than disease oriented.
18. 'World Health Organization' has Veterinary public health section in Division of Communicable Disease.

19. VPH section of WHO plays a liasoning role between public health and Veterinary profession worldwide.
20. World's largest non- governmental organization concerned with development of quality standards is WTO.
21. 'International Organisation for Standardisation' was established with the aim to facilitate international coordination and unification of industrial standards.
22. The WTO was formed on January 1, 1995, replacing the post-war multilateral trading order *i.e.* Technical Barrier on Trade (TBT).
23. WTO was established with the aim to enhance international sale of goods and services.
24. The ministerial conference in WTO comprises trade or commercial ministers of member countries.
25. A recent trade facilitation agreement of WTO called 'Bali Package' was accepted by all member countries on 7th December 2013.
26. The agreement of WTO that provides protection to plant health, animal health and human life from any risk is known as TBT.
27. The term 'codex alimentarius' is taken from a Latin word which means food code.
28. Codex Alimentarius commission was established by FAO and WHO for international food standards to guide food industry of the world and protect the health of consumer.
29. Risk analysis is well established for chemical hazards and now WHO and FAO are extending expertise towards microbiological hazards.
30. OIE was established in response to FMD outbreak in Europe.
31. OIE operates under international committee composed of delegates of member countries.
32. The 'National Institute of Veterinary Epidemiology and Disease Informatics' is situated at Chennai.
33. The 'National Institute of Communicable Diseases' (NICD) was established in 1934 at New Delhi.

34. NICD was established by the Government of India to expand and reorganize the activities of the 'Malaria Institute of India' (MII).

35. Central government plays more important role than state government in the wake of natural disaster.

36. Set of uniform standards envisaged to improve quality of health care delivery in the country is called Indian Public Health Standard.

37. 'Food Safety and Standard Authority of India' was established with the aim of laying down science based standards for article of food.

38. 'Food Safety and Standard Authority of India' was established in Sept. 2006 however Food safety and standard regulation was passed by Government of India in 2008.

39. Private public participation was a salient feature of PFA.

40. Multi level and multi departmental control in PFA act was brought under the arena of single line of control in FSSA act.

41. 'Bureau of Indian Standards' (BIS) was formerly known as ISO.

42. BIS is a statuary body working under the aegis of Ministry of health and family welfare.

43. BIS is a founder member of ISO and enquiry point for WTO.

44. Laboratory accreditation in India to get BIS certificate is done by 'National Accreditation Board for Testing and Calibration Laboratories'.

45. The training institute of BIS is known as 'National Institute of Training for Standardisation'.

46. 'National Institute of Training for Standardisation' is working from Lucknow, Uttar Pradesh.

47. International Commission for Microbiological Specification for Food has suggested three types of attribute sampling schemes for testing microbiological safety of foods.

48. In attribute sampling scheme, number of sample units from a lot that must be examined is denoted by 'n'.

49. In attribute sampling scheme, maximum allowable number of sample units that may exceed microbiological limits is denoted by 'c'.
50. The choice of sampling plan depends upon the seriousness of hazard and future conditions to which it is exposed.
51. If number of bacteria in all sample units does not exceed 'm' criterion, the results are considered satisfactory.
52. If number of bacteria in all sample units exceeds 'm' criterion, the sample is considered non- acceptable in 2 class plan and marginally acceptable in 3 class plan.
53. The microbiological criterion 'M' is applicable to 'two class plan'.
54. If number of bacteria in any of the sample units is at or above 'M', the sample is considered non- acceptable in 3 class sampling plan.
55. In '3 class sampling plan', value 'm' separates good quality from defective quality, while in '2 class sampling plan'; 'm' separates good quality from marginally acceptable.
56. HACCP and microbiological specifications are two excellent means of ensuring food safety and good keeping quality of food product.
57. HACCP is a systematic scientific approach to food safety that addresses physical, chemical and biological hazard as a means of prevention rather than finished product inspection.
58. Critical control point 1 in HACCP ensures that either hazard is minimized or controlled.
59. Critical control point 2 in HACCP ensures that hazard is completely eliminated.
60. A sample sent to food safety laboratory for microbiological and chemical examination should first be examined chemically.
61. *Cysticercus cellulose* and *Trichenella* are killed by freezing the meat.
62. Radurisation must be used along with refrigeration to enhance the shelf life of food product.
63. Water used in the cleaning and sanitizing of dairy plant should be moderately hard.

64. If the colony count/900 cm^2 area is 5000, it indicates good hygienic practices at dairy plant.

65. Satisfactory sanitation of dairy equipment is revealed by 10,000 CFU/900 cm^2 by swab method.

66. If none of the plate is showing 30-300 colonies, the plates nearest to 300 colonies should be considered for counting.

67. Membrane filtration method is preferred only when number of bacteria in a sample is very high.

68. Indicator organisms may or may not be responsible for the hazard.

69. University of Verment broth I and II are used as enrichment medium for *Yersinea enterocolitica.*

70. Alkaline peptone water with 3 per cent NaCl is a medium of choice for enrichment of *Vibrio parahaemolyticus.*

71. Cefsulodin irgasan novobiocin agar is the selective media for the isolation of *Yersinea enterocolitica* and shows red bull eye colony.

72. Mannital Egg Yolk Polymixin agar medium is used as selective medium for detection and determination of *Staphylococcus.*

73. Thiosulphate citrate bile salt agar is widely used as selective medium for isolation of all pathogenic vibrios.

74. *L. monocytogenes* is catalase positive, oxidase negative and motile at 20-30 °C.

75. The results of fermentation test are expressed as negative or positive for commercial sterility of canned food, when sample is incubated at 30°C/35°C for a period of 10 days.

76. Violet red bile agar medium is prepared by autoclaving at 121°C for 15 min.

77. The incubation temperature required to differentiate fecal coliforms from non-fecal coliforms is 55°C.

78. The antibiotics selected for use in food preservation should be other than those being used in the treatment of diseases.

79. UV rays affect only the outer surface of most irradiated foods and do not penetrate microorganism inside the food.

80. Positive air pressure should be maintained in microbiologically sensitive areas in a food plant to make ventilation more effective.
81. Metasilicate is very effective in holding the soil in suspension during the washing operation so that complete cleaning is possible.
82. The application of 'liquid smoke' to the outside of foods has little or no preservative effect as compared to 'wood smoke'.
83. Low dose radiation pasteurization with specific intent to eliminate a particular pathogen is called radicidation.
84. Ventilation opening should never be equipped with close fitting screen in food plant.
85. Washroom, lunchroom and change room should be adjacent to food processing area.
86. Potable, soft, hot and cold water should only be used in food industry.
87. Backflow protectors are necessary in plant at the source of water supply.
88. Proper drainage on the roof should be installed in food plant.
89. Doors in food plant should have smooth, absorbent surfaces and should be close fitting.
90. Equalization of the moisture to a desired level usually in the boxes is called sweating.
91. Slow freezing is better than quick freezing for preservation of food.
92. Organic matter in the form of serum, blood, pus, or fecal or lubricant material does not interfere with the antimicrobial activity of disinfectants.
93. Bacteria within the biofilms are more resistant to antimicrobials, freezing and drying than are the same bacteria in suspension.
94. Carl Von Linde developed a refrigeration process for the first time to preserve the food.
95. The concept of food safety is pertained to protecting the individual handling the agent; whereas concept of biosecurity is pertained to

protecting populations of human, animals and plants as well as environment.

96. Presence of Coliform in heat processed food is indicative of inadequate processing.

97. Poultry meat is major source of *Salmonella enteritidis* and *Campylobacter jejunni* infection as compared to red meat.

98. Nitrites can react with secondary or tertiary amines in food leading to formation of nitrosamine.

99. Heat processing is more effective if it is applied in dry form rather than in moist form.

100. The most important in food preservation is the lengthening the lag phase and phase of positive acceleration.

MATCHING TYPE QUESTIONS

Part A

Column – A		*Column – B*
1. Lag phase	(_)	a. Active growth phase
2. Log phase	(_)	b. Initial growth phase
3. Calvin W Schwabe	(_)	c. HACCP concept
4. H. E. Bauman	(_)	d. One health concept
5. Nicolas Appert	(_)	e. Cooling process
6. Car Von lynde	(_)	f. Canning process
7. Food hygiene	(_)	g. Bernard Bang
8. Disease control	(_)	h. Daniel Salmon
9. First vaccine for human	(_)	i. Louis Pasteur
10. First vaccine for animal	(_)	j. Edward Jenner

Part B

Column – A		*Column – B*
1. Saponifying agent	(__)	a. Irradiation
2. Wetting agent	(__)	b. Canning
3. Sequestering agent	(__)	c. *Klebsiella*
4. Cold sterilization	(__)	d. Polyphosphate
5. Radappertization	(__)	e. *Galionella*
6. Freezer burn	(__)	f. Strong alkali
7. Coliform	(__)	g. Calcium carbonate
8. Iron bacteria	(__)	h. Calcium sulphate.
9. Temporary hardness	(__)	i. Surfactant
10. Permanent hardness	(__)	j. Cold storage

Part C

Column – A		*Column – B*
1. PFA	(__)	a. Municipal Board
2. FSSA	(__)	b. Municipal Corporation
3. PD ADMAS	(__)	c. Jila Parishad
4. NICD	(__)	d. Panchayat Samiti
5. AIIH and PH	(__)	e. Bhopal
6. HSADL	(__)	f. Kolkata
7. BDO	(__)	g. Delhi
8. CEO	(__)	h. Bangluru
9. Mayer	(__)	i. Single authority
10. Chairman	(__)	j. Multiple authority

Part D

Column – A		*Column – B*
1. WTO	(__)	a. 1924
2. ISO	(__)	b. 1932
3. OIE	(__)	c. 1946
4. FSSAI	(__)	d. 1962
5. AIIH and PH	(__)	e. 1963
6. NICD	(__)	f. 1995
7. CAC	(__)	g. 2008
8. BSE	(__)	h. *Listeria monocytogenes*
9. EHEC O157	(__)	i. Unconventional agent
10. PALCAM	(__)	j. Conventional agent

ANSWERS

Multiple Choice Questions

1.(d)	2.(d)	3.(d)	4.(b)	5.(b)	6.(c)	7.(b)
8.(a)	9.(c)	10.(d)	11.(b)	12.(d)	13.(d)	14.(a)
15.(d)	16.(a)	17.(c)	18.(a)	19.(d)	20.(b)	21.(d)
22.(d)	23.(b)	24.(d)	25.(c)	26.(d)	27.(c)	28.(a)
29.(a)	30.(d)	31.(b)	32.(d)	33.(b)	34.(d)	35.(d)
36.(a)	37.(c)	38.(d)	39.(b)	40.(d)	41.(d)	42.(d)
43.(b)	44.(c)	45.(d)	46.(d)	47.(b)	48.(d)	49.(c)
50.(b)	51.(d)	52.(d)	53.(c)	54.(b)	55.(a)	56.(d)
57.(c)	58.(b)	59.(d)	60.(b)	61.(a)	62.(a)	63.(d)
64.(a)	65.(d)	66.(d)	67.(a)	68.(d)	69.(b)	70.(c)
71.(c)	72.(a)	73.(c)	74.(c)	75.(c)	76.(b)	77.(a)
78.(b)	79.(c)	80.(a)	81.(a)	82.(b)	83.(a)	84.(b)
85.(b)	86.(d)	87.(d)	88.(a)	89.(c)	90.(d)	91.(d)
92.(a)	93.(c)	94.(d)	95.(a)	96.(a)	97.(c)	98.(d)
99.(b)	100.(c)					

Fill in the Blanks

1. Goddess of health
2. Aesculapius
3. 'Sanitas', Cleanliness
4. Indus valley civilization
5. Mohanjodaro and Harrapa
6. Human medicine and Veterinary medicine
7. Community or group
8. Lyon, France
9. Centre for Disease Control (CDS) Atlanta and Prevention (CDC), Atlanta
10. 1975
11. Physical, mental, social well being
12. Field data
13. International Organisation for Standardisation
14. International Federation of National Standardizing Association (ISA) and United Nation Standards Coordinating Committee (UNSCC)

15. *isos*, equal
16. quality management
17. World Health Organization (WHO)
18. United States Department of Agriculture (USDA)
19. Food Safety and Inspection Service (FSIS)
20. Office International des Epizootics (OIE)
21. World Organization for Animal Health
22. Prof. Emmanuel Leclainche
23. Codex Alimentarius Commission (CAC)
24. Food safety
25. Animal Health
26. Five, Four, One
27. Four specialist
28. Fish diseases
29. International committee
30. International committee
31. OIE
32. IPPC, OIE, CAC
33. All India Institute of Hygiene and Public Health
34. PD-ADMAS
35. Veterinary Epidemiology and Disease Informatics
36. National Institute of High Security Animal Disease
37. 100
38. One lakh
39. Town area committees, municipal boards and corporation
40. Panchayati Raj
41. Gram Panchayat
42. Panchayat samiti
43. Zila Parishad
44. National Rural Health Mission
45. World Trade Organization (WTO)
46. General Agreement on Tariff and Trade
47. Transparency
48. Capacity building
49. Sanitary and Phytosanitary
50. SPS, TBT
51. 53rd, 2000
52. Farm to table
53. HACCP
54. Critical control point
55. Prevention of Food Adulteration
56. Food Safety and Standard Authority of India
57. Food Safety and Standard Act
58. International Commission on Microbiological Specification for Food
59. Highest limit

60. Threshold value
61. Sampling procedures, decision criteria
62. Presence or absence
63. Acceptable, unacceptable and marginally acceptable
64. Two class
65. Three class
66. Two class
67. m and M
68. Zero
69. 1-3
70. Indicators
71. 24h
72. 36h
73. 100 foot candles
74. 44-45°C
75. Robertson cooked Medium
76. Violet Red Bile agar
77. Fermentation test or Incubation test
78. Heketoen enteric agar
79. *L. monocytogenes*
80. MUG sorbitol agar
81. Wagasuma agar
82. National Institute of Cholera and Enteric Diseases at Kolkata
83. Sequestering
84. Nitrosamine
85. Blanching
86. BOD
87. Acidic
88. Sodium metasilicate
89. John Tyndall
90. Ehtylene and propylene oxide
91. Rise
92. 20 -70
93. Picowaved food
94. Trimethylamine
95. Lypophilic
96. SO_2
97. Scromboid
98. More than 80°C
99. Continuous chlorination
100. Z-value

Mark True/False

1. False
2. True
3. False
4. False
5. True
6. True
7. False
8. False
9. True
10. False
11. True
12. True
13. True
14. False
15. False
16. True
17. False
18. True
19. True
20. False
21. True
22. False
23. True
24. True
25. True
26. False
27. True
28. True
29. True
30. False
31. True
32. False
33. False
34. True
35. False
36. True
37. True
38. False
39. False
40. True
41. False
42. False
43. True
44. True
45. True
46. False
47. False
48. True
49. True
50. True
51. True
52. True
53. False
54. True
55. False
56. True
57. True
58. False
59. False
60. False
61. True
62. True
63. False
64. True
65. False
66. True
67. False
68. True
69. False
70. True
71. True
72. False
73. True
74. True
75. True
76. False
77. False
78. True
79. True
80. True
81. True
82. True
83. True
84. False
85. False
86. True
87. True
88. True
89. False
90. True
91. False
92. False
93. True
94. True
95. True
96. True
97. True
98. True
99. False
100. True

Matching Type Quetions

Part A

1. B
2. A
3. D
4. C
5. F
6. E
7. H
8. G
9. J
10. I

Part B

1. F
2. I
3. D
4. A
5. B
6. J
7. C
8. E
9. G
10. H

Part C

1. J
2. I
3. H
4. G
5. F
6. E
7. D
8. C
9. B
10. A

Part D

1. F
2. C
3. A
4. G
5. B
6. E
7. D
8. I
9. J
10. H

Chapter 2
Milk Hygiene

MULTIPLE CHOIE QUESTIONS

1. **The standard plate count of pasteurized milk/ml should not exceed:**
   (a) 20,000 (b) 40,000
   (c) 30,000 (d) 50,000
2. **The programme operation flood started in the year:**
   (a) 1960 (b) 1970
   (c) 1990 (c) 1996
3. **The pH of normal cow milk is:**
   (a) 7.8 (b) 4.2
   (c) 6.6 (d) 7.5
4. **In HTST method of pasteurization, milk is exposed to:**
   (a) 72°C (b) 12 0°C
   (c) 62.3°C (d) 100°C
5. **The heating temperature used in LTLT/Batch holder method is:**
   (a) 61.5°C (b) 62.8°C
   (c) 63.5°C (d) 64.5°C

6. **Turbidity test is done for:**
   (a) Pasteurized milk (b) Sterilized milk
   (c) Adulterated milk (d) Contaminated milk

7. **'Hansa test' is done to check adulteration of cow milk with:**
   (a) Goat milk (b) Mare milk
   (c) Buffalo milk (d) Ewe milk

8. **MBR test is done to adjudge the ______ of milk:**
   (a) Bacteriological quality (b) Organoleptic quality
   (c) Physical quality (d) Chemical quality

9. **Phage inhibiting media is deficient in:**
   (a) Calcium (b) Mgnesium
   (c) Zinc (d) Iron

10. **The milk which is low in bacterial load, free from pathogen, chemical residues or abnormal secretion is called:**
    (a) Clean milk (b) Wholesome milk
    (c) Pure milk (d) Sterilized milk

11. **All the following organism belong to coliform group except:**
    (a) E. coli (b) *Klebsiella*
    (c) Proteus (d) *Enterobacter*

12. **The burnt flavor in milk is caused by:**
    (a) Overheating
    (b) *Streptococcus lactis* var. *maltigenes*
    (c) Both of above
    (d) None of above

13. **The example of the test used to diagnose *Brucellosis* in a milch herd is:**
    (a) MBR (b) MAT
    (c) MRT (d) CAMP

14. Milk allergy is caused by:

(a) Milk Sugar
(b) Bacterial Toxin
(c) Milk Protein
(d) Inhibitory Factor

15. Surface Ropiness in milk is caused by:

(a) *Enterobacter aerogenes*
(b) *E.coli*
(c) *Klebsiella oxytoca*
(d) *Alkaligens viscolactis*

16. The detergent used to saponify fat are basically:

(a) Strong acid
(c) Strong alkali
(b) Weak acid
(d) Weak alkali

17. The milk and milk product order is a regulatory order of Govt. of India for control of _______ of milk and milk product:

(a) Production
(b) Supply
(c) Distribution
(d) All of above

18. Tick borne encephalitis is transmitted through _______ milk:

(a) Cattle
(b) Goat
(c) Sheep
(d) Mare

19. The strains of *Clostridium perfringens* causing gastroenteritis in human produce:

(a) Alpha toxin
(b) Epsilon toxin
(c) Beta toxin
(d) Iota toxin

20. Normal contaminants that are inhibitory to *Staphylococci* in milk are :

(a) Proteolytic bacteria
(b) Lactic acid bacteria
(c) Butyric acid bacteria
(d) Lipolytic bacteria

21. *E. coli* producing infantile diarrhoea in children fed with unheated milk are:

(a) EPEC
(b) EIEC
(c) ETEC
(d) EHEC

22. All the following are thermoduric organism except one:

(a) *Corynebacterium* (b) Microbacterium

(c) *Flavobacterium* (d) *Micrococci*

23. Bifidus factor, a natural inhibitory substance is found in:

(a) Bovine milk (b) Human milk

(c) Goat milk (d) Mare milk

24. A classical example of milk borne disease that causes intoxication is:

(a) Brucellosis (b) Listeriosis

(c) Staphylococcosis (d) Camplobacteriosis

25. Lactose content is maximum in the milk of:

(a) Cattle (b) Goat

(c) Sheep (d) Human

26. The bacteria that become problematic, if milk is held in pasteurizer for long time are:

(a) Psychrophilic (b) Thermoduric

(c) Thermophilic (d) Psychrotrophic

27. Energy value of cow milk is:

(a) 75 calorie/100g (b) 95 calorie/100g

(c) 85 calorie/100g (d) 100 calorie/100g

28. As per BIS, Yeast and mold count is of great significance for quality assurance of:

(a) Butter (b) Ice cream

(c) Cream (d) Milk Powder

29. Water content is maximum in the milk of:

(a) Cattle (b) Goat

(c) Sheep (d) Human

30. Which of the following is psychrophilic in nature?

(a) Alkaligens (b) Pseudomonas

(c) Achromobacter (d) All of above

31. The iron binding protein found in milk is:

(a) Lactoferrin (b) Siderophore

(c) Transferrin (d) Lactoglobulin

32. Bitter flavour and taste of milk is caused by:

(a) Proteolytic bacteria (b) Lipolytic bacteria

(c) Both of the above (d) None of the above

33. Ropiness in milk is caused by:

(a) *Enterobacter aerogenes* (b) *E. coli*

(c) *Klebsiella oxytoca* (d) All of the above

34. Surface taint or rabbito in unsalted butter is caused by:

(a) *Pseudomonas putrifaciens* (b) *Aeromonas hydrophil*

(c) Mold (d) Yeast

35. The chief gas former in raw milk are:

(a) *Clostridium* (b) *Coliform*

(c) *Bacillus* (d) All of the above

36. Aroma producing organism of milk belongs to the genus:

(a) *Streptococcus* (b) *Leuconostoc*

(c) Both of the above (d) None of the above

37. Swelling of the can is caused by gas forming anaerobic spore former *i.e.*

(a) *Clostridium* spp. (b) *Bacillus* spp.

(c) *Micrococci* (d) *Streptococci*

38. Coagulation of milk in sealed can may be blamed to all the following organism except:

(a) *Bacillus cereus* (b) *Bacillus subtilis*

(c) *Bacillus megaterium* (d) *Streptococci*

39. Sweet curdling in pasteurized milk is caused by:

(a) *Proteus* sp. (b) *Pseudomonas* sp

(c) *Flavobacterium* sp. (d) *Bacillus cereus*

40. Blue color in milk is caused by:

(a) *Ps. putrifaciens* (b) *Ps. synxantha*

(c) *Ps. fragi* (d) *Ps. syncyanea*

41. Which of the following bacterium is acid proteolytic in nature?

(a) *Bacillus cereus*

(b) *Strept. faecalis var. liquifaciens*

(c) *Proteus vulgaris*

(d) *Clostridium sporogenes*

42. Unhygienic condition of equipment may impart carbolic taint to milk which is caused by:

(a) *Bacillus subtilis* (b) *Bacillus circulans*

(c) *Bacillus cereus* (d) *Bacillus coagulans*

43. All the following organisms are thermoduric except one:

(a) *Micrococci* (b) *Flavobacterium*

(c) *Microbacterium* (d) *Streptococci*

44. The intoxication caused by boiled milk left at room temperature, is associated with:

(a) *Staphylococcus aureus* (b) *Vibrio cholerae*

(c) *Clostridium botulinum* (d) *E. coli*

45. The presence of which organism is indicative of inefficient sterilization.

(a) *Bacillus stearothermophyllus* (b) *Bacillus subtilis*

(c) Both of above (d) None of above

46. The milk borne viral disease(s) which can be transmitted by infected handlers is/are

(a) Polio (b) Coxsackie virus

(C) Hepatitis (d) All of above

47. Milk borne pathogen that survives and multiplies in refrigerated products and associated with encephalitis, abortion and conjunctivitis in man, is

(a) *Listeria* (b) *Corynebacterium*

(c) *Leptospira* (d) *Campylobacter*

48. The Lactobacilli which is not homofermentative:

(a) *L. acidophilus.* (b) *L. plantarum*

(c) *L. fermentum* (d) *L. bulgaricus*

49. Bacteria that survive pasteurization temperature but do not multiply are called:

(a) Thermostable (b) Thermophilic

(c) Thermoduric (d) Thermoresistant

50. Scarlet fever is caused by:

(a) *Corynebacterium* (b) *Coxsackie* virus

(c) *Streptococci* (d) *Bacillus*

51. Condition(s) necessary for outbreaks of *Clostridium perfringens* through contaminated cooked food is/are:

(a) Holding temp. <60 °C (b) Reduced condition

(c) Inadequate cooling (d) All of above

52. Which of the following organism produces most potent neurotoxin?

(a) *Cl. perfringen* (b) *Cl. tetani*

(c) *Cl. botulinum* (d) *Cl. butyricum*

53. Which of the following BIS standard is used for sterilized milk?

(a) Standard plate count (b) Yeast and mold count

(b) Coliform count (d) Spore count

54. Rat bite fever is caused by:

(a) *Streptococcus moniliformis* (b) *Streptococcus agalactiae*

(c) *Streptococcus pyogenes* (d) *Streptococcus faecalis*

55. The bacterium whose toxin is most potent, is:

(a) *Staphylococcus aureus* (b) *E. coli*

(c) *Bacillus cereus* (d) *Cl. botulinum*

56. The test exclusively used for testing efficiency of sterilization of milk is:

(a) Coliform test (b) Turbidity test

(c) Hotis test (d) Phosphatase test

57. The optimum temperature required for the growth of psychotroph is:

(a) 25-30°C (b) 10-15°C

(c) 15-20°C (d) 7-10°C

58. Spoilage of pasteurized milk held at refrigerated temperature is mainly caused by:

(a) Psychrophilic organism (b) Psychotrophic organism

(c) Thermoduric organism (d) Thermophilic organism

59. Acid proteolysis of milk causes shrunken curd with lots of whey and this change is brought about by:

(a) *Micrococcus* sp. (b) *Bacillus* sp.

(c) Enterococci (d) All of above

60. 'AGMARK' certification is mainly applied for which dairy product:

(a) Ghee (b) Butter

(c) Fat spread (d) All of above

61. Growth of which acid producer commences first in raw milk at 10-37°C:

(a) *Streptococcus lactis* (b) *Coliform*

(c) *Lactobacilli* (d) *Micrococci*

62. The process of skimming in milk is accomplished by:

(a) Lowering of fat (b) Addition of water

(c) Removal of fat (d) All of above

63. The dye reduction time depends upon______ of bacteria:

(a) Number (b) Metabolic activity

(c) Type (d) All of above

64. Which of the following BIS standard is incorrect for pasteurized milk?

(a) MBR time-5hr

(b) Alkaline phophatase-negative

(c) SPC- not more than 30,000cfu/ml

(d) Coliform-absent in1:10 dilution

65. Rancidity in milk and milk product is caused by:

(a) Oxidation of fat (b) Hydrolysis of fat

(c) Both of above (d) None of above

66. The quality of water used in hygiene of dairy plant should be:

(a) Potable (b) Hard

(c) Chlorinated (d) All of above

67. Washing of teat and udder should be carried out with______ solution of potassium permagnate:

(a) 1 per cent (b) 3 per cent

(c) 2 per cent (d) 10 per cent

68. The concentration of all the following constituents decreases in mastitic milk except:

(a) Casein (b) Fat

(c) Lactose (d) Chloride

69. The species having 89.1 per cent (highest) of water in milk is:

(a) Human (b) Goat

(c) Mare (d) Cow

70. The species having highest 8.6 per cent of fat in milk is:

(a) Buffalo (b) Sheep

(c) Yak (d) Cow

71. The stain used for direct microscopic count to stain the milk smear is:

(a) Lieshman's stain (b) *Newman's Lampert stain*

(c) Sellar's stain (d) Lactophenol cotton blue

72. Verghese Kurien is credited for the foundation of:

(a) AMUL (b) NDDB

(c) IRMA (d) All of above

73. Reference strain used for detection of antibiotic residues in milk by dye reduction test is:

(a) *Bacillus stearothermophilus* (b) *Streptococcus thermophilus*

(c) *Lactobacillus thermophilus* (d) *Sarcinea lutea*

74. The incubation period of staphylococcal food poisoning ranges between:

(a) 2-6 hrs (c) 8-12 hrs

(b) 6-8 hrs (d) 12-24 hrs

75. The incubation temperature used to differentiate fecal coliform from non-fecal coliform is :

(a) 44°C (b) 25°C

(c) 37°C (d) 15°C

76. The natural acidity of milk is because of:

(a) Acid phosphate (b) Citrate

(c) Casein (d) All of above

77. All the following elements are major constituent of milk except:

(a) Iron (b) Potassium

(c) Sodium (d) Magnesium

78. The critical control point in HACCP system means:

(a) Any location (b) Any practice

(c) Any process (d) All of above

79. The term hazard in HACCP systems is used to refer any ______ of microorganism (biological hazards):

(a) Unacceptable contamination (b) Growth

(b) Survival (d) All of above

80. The presence of hydrogen peroxide in milk is detected by adding para-phenyl diamine which gives:

(a) Red color (b) Yellow color

(c) Violate color (d) Blue color

81. The standard plate count of 5-10 lacs/ml denotes______ quality of raw milk:

(a) Excellent (b) Fair

(c) Good (d) Poor

82. Which method is the best to enhance keeping quality of milk?

(a) LTLT (b) HTST

(c) UHT-ST (d) Boiling

83. Which criterion is not true to meet the requirement of wholesome milk?

(a) Free from bacterial load

(b) Free from antibiotic residue

(c) Free from chemical residue

(d) Free from adulteration

84. How much milk sample is drawn from bulk container for microbiological analysis?

(a) 5 ml (b) 15 ml

(c) 25 ml (d) 100 ml

85. All the following tests are used to diagnose mastitis except

(a) Strip cup test (b) CMT test

(c) CAMP test (d) White side test

86. All the following tests are placed in the category of rapid platform test except:

(a) Organoleptic test (b) Alcohol test

(c) Clot on boiling (d) Direct microscopic count

87. All the following organism are responsible for yellow coloration in milk except:

(a) *Ps. aerugenosa* (b) *Sarcinea lutea*

(c) *Ps. synxantha* (d) *Mycobacterium flavum*

88. Which of the following is known as dairy worker fever?

(a) Leptospirosis (b) Brucellosis

(c) Listeriosis (d) Tuberculosis

89. The founder chairperson of 'National Dairy Development Board' was:

(a) Verghese Kurien (b) Sardar Vallabh Bhai Patel

(c) Tribhuvan Das (d) Amrita Patel

90. Fluctuating fever, headache, night sweats with peculiar odour, pain in joints and muscle are the characteristics of:

(a) Undulant fever (b) Typhoid fever

(c) Q fever (d) Scarlet fever

91. As per ICMSF, *Coxiella burnetti* has been categorized as______ type of microbiological hazard:

(a) Severe (b) Moderate

(c) Low (d) None of above

92. All the following pathogens have been placed in the category of severe hazard as per ICMSF except:

(a) *Salmonella typhi* (b) *Salmonella typhimurium*

(c) *Salmonella paratyphi* (d) *Shiegella dysenteriae*

93. The concept of HACCP was for the first time introduced by:

(a) H.E. Bauman (b) James Jay

(c) Edwards and Ewing (d) Charles Badwin

94. All the following pathogens have been placed in the category of severe hazard as per ICMSF except:

(a) *Clostridium botulinum* (b) *Vibrio cholerae*

(c) *Brucella melitensis* (d) *Staphylococcus aureus*

95. At higher temperature (37-50 °C), which one will produce more acid?

(a) *Streptococcus lactis* (b) *Lactobacillus bulgaricus*

(c) *Streptococcus thermophilus* (d) *Streptococcus faecalis*

96. The major source of *Bacillus cereus* in milk is/are:

(a) Infected animal (b) Soil

(c) Contaminated utensils (d) All of above

97. The pathogenic organism that originate from handlers at source and produce most heat stable toxins:

(a) *Staphylococcus aureus* (b) Entertoxigenic E. coli

(c) *Bacillus cereus* (d) All of above

98. 'Kefir' is an acidic alcoholic fermented product which is prepared from milk of:

(a) Cow (b) Sheep

(c) Goat (d) All of above

99. 'Kumiss' is an acidic alcoholic fermented product which is prepared from milk of:

(a) Cow (b) Sheep

(c) Goat (d) Mare

100. Bloody milk without apparent swelling of udder, abortion along with fever, anemia, icterus, haemoglobinuria are the characteristics of :

(a) *Leptospirosis* (b) *Listeriosis*

(c) *Salmonellosis* (d) *Crptococcosis*

FILL IN THE BLANKS

1. The titrable acidity of normal milk ranges between _______.
2. Milk with acidity more than _______ clots on boiling.
3. The best test, which is used for determining sanitary quality of milk, is _______ because it counts only viable bacteria.
4. For determining the total bacterial count of milk, _______ test is conducted.
5. A microscopic factor of _______ is considered important during bacterial cell and leukocyte counting of the milk sample.
6. Milk with alkaline pH is suitable for the growth of _______.
7. The total cell count (TVC) of milk obtained from healthy udder ranges from _______.
8. If the animal is suffering from mastitis, _______ cell count will increase.
9. _______ and _______ are called leucoform dyes because their color changes with the decrease in redox potential.
10. The enzyme bacterial _______ catalyses oxidation reduction in milk and reduces the color of dye.

11. The change in the color of redox dyes is brought about by ______ and ______ (cells) present in milk.
12. Methylene blue reduction time of pasteurized milk should be______.
13. The standard plate count of pasteurized milk should not exceed _______.
14. A test performed in milk processing plant to test the efficiency of pasteurization is called ______.
15. The enzyme which is present in improperly pasteurized milk is _______.
16. In phosphatase test, ______ is used as substrate.
17. The legislation that prescribes provision for orderly development of Indian dairy industry is ______.
18. Microorganisms found in milk are broadly classified in two categories 1. ______ 2. ______.
19. Based on growth temperature, microorganisms found in milk are classified into three categories 1. ______ 2. ______ 3.______.
20. Tallow flavor in milk is caused by oxidation of ______fatty acid.
21. The organism that imparts burnt flavour to milk is ______.
22. Bacillus ______is associated with carbolic taint in milk.
23. The oxidation and hydrolysis of milk fat by lipolytic bacteria produces _______.
24. Defective change that causes curdling of milk without production of acid is called as ______.
25. Sweet curdling is coagulation of milk proteins without acid production by ______ like enzyme.
26. Surface ropiness in milk is caused by______
27. The major source of OCL pesticide residue in milk is ______ and _______.
28. Butter contains ______ proportion of Chlorinated hydrocarbon (DDT) residue than liquid milk.

29. An average withdrawal period followed for milk obtained from antibiotic treated cow must be at least _______.

30. Radionuclide, which was reported for the first time to be present in milk, was _______.

31. Starter failure in dairy industry is caused by_______.

32. Hotis test is used to diagnose mastitis caused by _______.

33. Use of _______ (hormone) for increasing the milk yield increases the susceptibility of udder for mastitis.

34. Major environmental contaminants present in milk produced under poor hygienic condition at dairy farm are _______ in nature.

35. The optimum temperature required for the growth of Psychrotroph is_______.

36. There is _______ percent loss in creamy layer after pasteurization.

37. Sweet curdling of pasteurized milk is caused by_______ (organism).

38. The bacteria that survive at pasteurization temperature but don't multiply are called _______.

39. Milk can be stored for _______ hrs at room temperature, immediately after milking.

40. The pH of normal milk ranges between_______.

41. Overheating of milk at high temperature imparts cooked flavour due to_______ compound.

42. The tallow flavour, bitter taste and rancidity in milk is caused by_______

43. Pasteurization in milk was invented by_______

44. The indicator organism for pasteurization is_______.

45. The LTLT method of pasteurization is also known as _______.

46. Keeping quality of pasteurized milk at 4°C is_______

47. The sub-temperature milk is diverted back to float controlled balance tank by _______ in HTST method.

48. The incoming milk is heated by outgoing pasteurized milk in _______ section in a pasteurization plant.

49. UHT method involves heating of milk at_______ temperature for_______ time.

50. Removal of microorganism from milk under centrifugal force is known as _______.
51. Heating of milk by direct steam under pressure is known as _______
52. Heating of milk at 137°C for a fraction of second is called as _______
53. Shelf-life of aseptically packed sterilized milk is_______ at room temperature.
54. Name the mesophilic index organism which is destroyed by UHT processing method _______.
55. Name the thermophilic index organism which is destroyed by UHT processing method is _______.
56. The milk lactose and amino acid lysine react with each other, if the milk is heated at high temperature for long time. This is called as _______
57. In maillard reaction, progressive inactivation of the _______ (amino acid) may take place due to prolong holding of sterilized milk at high temperature.
58. The test used to determine bacteriological quality of sterilized milk is _______.
59. The test used to determine efficiency of sterilization is called _______.
60. The sterility test of UHT processed milk is carried out by incubating the sample at 30°C for_______.
61. The temperature of lukewarm water used for pre rinsing of dairy equipments should not be more than _______.
62. The wall of dairy plant should be tiled up to the height of_______.
63. The hardness of water used for washing and sanitization purpose in dairy plant should not be more than _______.
64. A minimum of _______ distance is necessary between the bottom of equipment and floor of dairy plant for proper cleaning.
65. No objection certificate should be obtained from _______ for discharge of waste or effluent of dairy plant.
66. Commonly used sanitizer in dairy industry is _______.

67. The permissible limit of H_2O_2 in milk should be______ ppm as per the recommendation of FAO.

68. Commonly used preservative in milk is ______.

69. The chemical used to detect urea adulteration in milk is 1 per cent _______.

70. The reagent used to detect presence of neutralizer in milk is ______.

71. The test used to detect adulteration of starch in milk is ______.

72. Skimming refers to the removal or lowering of ______ from milk.

73. Skimming causes ______ in specific gravity.

74. The medium which can be used to enumerate *Staphylococci* in milk product is ______ medium.

75. The medium which can be used to enumerate *Coliform* in milk and milk product is called______ medium.

76. PALCAM agar medium is used for isolation of______ from milk product.

77. For isolating *Mycobacterium tuberculosis* from milk,______ culture medium is used.

78. Milk having penicillin residues may cause ______ in a sensitive individual.

79. The active principle of snake root poisoning that may occur through milk is ______.

80. Consumption of milk contaminated with rat saliva causes ______.

81. Name two emerging pathogenic bacteria having importance in refrigerated milk products 1. ______ 2. ______.

82. Bacterium that originate from dirty environment and produces diarrhoeal and emetic syndrome is______.

83. Emetic syndrome in *Bacillus cereus* toxicity is caused by ______ toxin.

84. The example of a rickettsial disease transmitted by milk is ______.

85. A tick borne viral disease which is also transmitted by ingestion of goat milk is ______.

86. A bacterium that causes milk borne toxi-infection is _______.

87. Milk contaminated with rat urine may cause _______.

88. The chief site of predilection for *Brucella* in non-pregnant cow is _______ and supramammary gland.

89. A serological test performed in milk to detect brucellosis in dairy herd is called _______.

90. Infantile diarrhoea through fecally contaminated milk is caused by _______.

91. Scarlet fever, a classical example of milk borne infection, is caused by_______.

92. Contamination of Infectious Hepatitis and Polio virus in milk mainly comes from _______.

93. The main organ affected in aflatoxicosis is _______.

94. The major sources of *Vibrio cholerae* in milk are _______ and _______.

95. The enzyme _______ is naturally present in milk and extends the shelf-life of fresh milk.

96. The essential components of LP system are lactoperoxidase, _______ and _______.

97. Thiocynate acts as _______ and H_2O_2 acts as _______ in LP system.

98. Germicidal property of milk is destroyed by heating at _______ for 30 min.

99. The test organism used by IDF for detection of antibiotic residues in milk by microbial inhibition test, is _______.

100. Limulus lysate is used for detection of bacterial _______ of Gram negative bacteria.

MARK TRUE/FALSE

1. *Bacillus circulans* survives at lower temperature in milk and gives extremely bitter taste.
2. Pathogenic bacteria multiply better in raw milk than in boiled milk at room temperature.
3. Chloride content of milk is increased beyond the critical value of 0.17 per cent, when mastitis is present.
4. *Mycobacterium tuberculosis* is always absent in pasteurized milk.
5. The pour plate method can be used to count the total number of bacteria present in milk.
6. Tetra-thionate broth is the only enrichment medium which can be used to isolate Salmonellae from milk.
7. There is inactivation of essential fatty acids by maillard's reaction when sterilized milk is stored for longer duration.
8. Milk containing antibiotic residues may develop antibiotic resistance and GI tract disturbance in human.
9. *Staphylococcus aureus* produces a poisonous substance in warm milk food. It is called endotoxin.
10. Direct microscopic count cannot be used to judge the quality of pasteurized milk.
11. FMD virus is not shed in the milk of affected animal.
12. The antibiotics present in milk are inactivated after pasteurization.
13. Oil based antibiotics remain in milk for longer time.
14. Presence of coliform in pasteurized milk indicates pre-processing contamination.
15. Rejection of fore milk is necessary for quality control test.
16. Cream is likely to contain higher proportion of microorganism than most lots of milk.

17. *Brucella* and *Mycobacterium* do not rapidly multiply in raw milk.
18. The starter culture for yoghurt consists of *Streptococcus lactis* and *Lactobacillus delbruckii.*
19. Most strains of phages are inactivated at normal pasteurization temperature.
20. Sri Lal Bahadur Shastri laid down the foundation of Anand Milk Union Limited.
21. *Lactobacilli* generally predominate in sour dahi, while *Streptococci* predominate in sweet dahi.
22. *Pseudomonas* and *Flavobacterium* are major spoilage organism in pasteurized milk stored at low temperature.
23. Ultra high temperature treated milk is as good as sterilized milk from microbiological point of view.
24. There is around 50 per cent loss in creamy layer after pasteurization.
25. Aseptically packed sterilized milk can be kept for month at room temperature.
26. Aromatic flavour in milk is a desirable change.
27. Normal milk is usually deficient in urea and chloride.
28. Presently, the indicator organism for pasteurization is *Mycobacterium tuberculosis*.
29. L. P. system is naturally found antimicrobial system in human milk.
30. The toxin produced by *Staphylococus aureus* is heat labile.
31. Surface taint or rabbito in unsalted butter is caused by *Pseudomonas fragi*.
32. Prolong keeping of milk in pasteurizer increases the problem of thermophiles.
33. Heating of milk at a temperature of 100°C or more for 2-3 minutes is called sterilization.
34. Milk produced from diseased udder may coagulate more rapidly than the milk produced by healthy udder.
35. Immunoglobulin A and G are found in milk.
36. Use of hydrogen peroxide is permissible in milk as per PFA, Act.

37. Milk allergy is caused by milk protein rather than toxins found in milk.
38. Chances of milk stone formation are more in LTLT method.
39. Installation of quality management system laid down in ISO:14000 series is essential for international trade of dairy product.
40. Coliform and phosphatase tests are used to determine the efficiency of pasteurization.
41. MBR test determine the exact number of bacteria in milk.
42. The concept of organized dairy farming in India originated from Anand District, Gujarat.
43. The national agency concerned with control of export and import of milk is NDDB.
44. As per ICMR, per capita availability of milk in India should be 263 gram/day.
45. Kefir is an acidic alcoholic fermented product of mare milk.
46. All the bacterial toxins are inactivated at pasteurization temperature.
47. The quality standards for milk and milk products in India are mainly confined to determination of chemical adulterants.
48. Vacreation of cream helps to remove off flavour.
49. Yeast and mold are most common contaminants in butter and yoghurt.
50. Formation of milk stone in pasteurizer is mainly associated with use of soft water.
51. In case of faulty or inefficient pasteurization, a red coloured compound p-nitrophenol is formed as a result of enzyme-substrate reaction.
52. We should never collect composite sample for testing of mastitis in dairy herd.
53. Bacteriophages can remain viable for very long time in dried up preparations and utensil.
54. Presence of thermophile in pasteurized milk is indicative of unhygienic condition at farm.

55. The milk protein casein is known as whey protein.
56. Removal of microorganism under centrifugal force is known as separation.
57. There are chances of formation of milk stone in pasteurizer in HTST method.
58. The spores of anthrax bacilli are not destroyed at usual sterilization process *i.e.,* 100°C for 10 min.
59. Acid detergent helps to remove milk stone and water scale.
60. Live attenuated spore vaccine of anthrax can be used in human being.
61. *Lactobacilli* are usually less in number than *Streptococci* but produce more acidity.
62. Coliform should be absent in pasteurized milk in 1:100 dilution as per BIS standards.
63. Problem of bacteriophage in dairy industry can be solved either by (phage intensive medium) mixed culture or rotation of culture.
64. Staphlylococcal intoxications are mainly caused by boiled milk rather than raw milk kept at ambient temperature.
65. Cheese may be subjected to spoilage during ripening by lactate fermenting *Clostridium* which may alter its texture and flavour.
66. The formation of pink colored ring on the top of milk sample in milk ring test is observed after 24 hour incubation at 37°C.
67. A serological test which is used for screening of *Brucella* positive animals in a herd is called RBPT.
68. The thermophilic organism which is destroyed by UHT processing method and used as index organism to determine time and temperature combination is *Bacillus megaterium.*
69. BIS has set a very lenient standard of less than 5 spores per ml of sterilized milk.
70. Sardar Vallabh Bhai Patel laid down the foundation of Anand Milk Union Limited.
71. Most of the fermented milks are tested for coliform and yeast and mold which are the most common contaminant in milk.

72. Undulent fever, a classical example of milk borne disease is characterized by biphasic fever, abortion, infertility, muscle weakness, arthritis and night sweats in man.

73. The aromatic flavor in milk is caused by a compound diaetyl produced as a result of oxidation of glucose.

74. The Baird Parker medium is used to determine faecal *Streptococci* in milk.

75. Milk is a clean white lacteal secretion of mammary gland excluding 5 days before and 15 days after calving.

76. Alcohol test can be used to determine acidity as well as neutralizers in milk.

77. Presence of fine and uniform size flakes in milk after addition of alcohol indicates absence of neutralizer, however bigger size flakes indicate presence of neutralizer.

78. The indirect tests used to determine microbiological quality of milk are based upon presence or absence of bacteria in milk.

79. Milk is an excellent source of calcium and phosphorus while iron and copper are present in traces.

80. The redox potential shows decline in milk, as more and more oxygen is consumed.

81. Food poisoning strains of *Clostridium perfringens* are mostly heat resistant and type A and C are more pathogenic than others for human being.

82. Bacteriophages are destroyed by boiling but survive ordinary pasteurization temperature.

83. Many proteolytic bacteria can produce acid fermentation in milk but only when conditions are unfavorable for lactics.

84. *Clostridium* spp. can produce butyric acid in milk under the conditions that prevent or inhibit lactics.

85. Milk held at freezing temperature is more prone to spoilage by proteolytic bacteria.

86. Operation flood programme of India completed in three phases in 1996.

87. The shelf life of UHT milk is six month at 4° C.

88. The shelf life of HTST milk at 4.4 to 7.2° C is 1-2 days.

89. The presence of psychrophilic organism in pasteurized milk may indicate contamination due to polluted water used in rinsing the equipment.

90. The spoilage organisms are unable to survive in yoghurt due to high acidity.

91. Resazurin test can be placed in the category of rapid platform test.

92. The time duration for taking observation in resazurin test is 30 min.

93. The key feature of Milk and Milk Product Order is compulsory registration of dairy farmers.

94. The milk obtained from healthy udder consists of approximately 10 per cent polymorphonuclear (PMN) cells while milk from infected udder consists of 90 per cent PMNs of total cell count.

95. Cleaning in place is practiced in bigger dairies while manual cleaning is practiced in small dairies.

96. Salted butter is less likely to support microbial growth than unsalted butter.

97. Churn is the main source of contamination in butter, so it should be sanitized with 200 mg/l chlorine solution prior to use.

98. If the average colony count/milk bottle is less than 800, it indicates satisfactory hygienic status.

99. Assessment of dairy plant or equipment sanitation is done by colony count/900 sq. cm. area.

100. A case of mastitis can be diagnosed by Direct Microscopic count of milk smear.

MATCHING TYPE QUESTIONS

Part A

Column – A		Column – B
1. Blue milk	(__)	a. *Staphylococus aureus*
2. Yellow milk	(__)	b. *Streptococcus lactis* var. *maltigenes*
3. Red milk	(__)	c. *Streptococcus agalacteiae*
4. Brown milk	(__)	d. *Streptococcus thermophilus*
5. Musty flavour	(__)	e. *Clostridium perfringens*
6. Intoxication	(__)	f. *Actinomycetes*
7. Toxi infection	(__)	g. *Ps. putrefaciens*
8. Pyogenic gp	(__)	h. *Serratia marcescens*
9. Viridans gp	(__)	i. *Ps. synxantha*
10. Burnt flavour	(__)	j. *Ps. syncyanea*

Part B

Column – A		Column – B
1. Lactoperoxidase	(__)	a. Oxidation of unsaturated fatty acid
2. Bifidus factor	(__)	b. Oxidation of sugar
3. Aromatic flavour	(__)	c. Clarification of milk
4. Rancid flavour	(__)	d. Break up fat globule
5. Ropiness	(__)	e. *Streptococcus pyogenes*
6. Scarlet fever	(__)	f. Bovine milk
7. Undulent fever	(__)	g. Human milk
8. Q fever	(__)	h. *Alkaligens viscolactis*
9. Bactofugation	(__)	i. Malta fever
10. Homogenization	(__)	j. Abattoir fever

Part C

Column – A		Column – B
1. Aromatic flavor	(__)	a. *Psuedomonas fragi*
2. Clean Acidic flavor	(__)	b. *Streptococcus lactis* var. *maltigenes*
3. Tallow flavor	(__)	c. *Bacillus coagulans*
4. Fruity flavor	(__)	d. *Aeromonas*
5. Musty flavor	(__)	e. *Proteolyitc bacteria*
6. Burnt flavor	(__)	f. *Actinomycetes*
7. Bitter flavour	(__)	g. *Lipolytic bacteria*
8. Sharp acidic flavour	(__)	h. *Coliform*
9. Fishiness	(__)	i. *Streptococcus lactis*
10. Phenolic odour	(__)	j. *Leuconostoc*

Part D

Column – A		Column – B
1. Caramel	(__)	a. Psychrophilic
2. *Bacillus thermoliquifaciens*	(__)	b. Carbolic odour
3. *Bacillus subtilis*	(__)	c. Burnt flavor
4. *Bacillus circulans*	(__)	d. Thermophilic
5. *Pseudomonas fragi*	(__)	e. Thermoduric
6. Acid detergent	(__)	f. Rosailic acid test
7. Strong alkali	(__)	g. Iodine test
8. Neutralizer	(__)	i. Preservative
9. Starch	(__)	j. Fat
10. Formalin	(__)	k. Milk stone

Part E

Column – A		Column – B
1. Lactoperoxidase	(__)	a. Flowcytometer
2. Lysozyme	(__)	b. Gerber's butyrometer
3. Staphylococcal toxin	(__)	c. Lactometer
4. *E. coli* toxin	(__)	d. Burette
5. Specific gravity	(__)	e. Bovine milk
6. Fat per cent	(__)	f. Human milk
7. Cell analysis	(__)	g. Exotoxin
8. Titrable acidity	(__)	h. Endotoxin
9. Human botulism	(__)	i. Type A,B,E
10. Animal botulism	(__)	j. Type C, D

Part F

Column – A		Column – B
1. Specific gravity of milk fat	(__)	a. Staphlococcal toxin
2. Specific gravity of SNF	(__)	b. *Vibrio parahaemolyticus* toxin
3. Specific gravity of water	(__)	c. *Clostridium perfringens* enterotoxin
4. Baudouin test	(__)	d. Anthrax
5. Babcock test	(__)	e. Brucellosis
6. Kitten test	(__)	f. 0.93 per cent
7. Kanagawa test	(__)	g. 1.614 per cent
8. Naglar's reaction	(__)	h. 1.0 per cent
9. Ascoli's test	(__)	i. Adulteration in ghee
10. Abortus bang ring test	(__)	j. Fat content

ANSWERS

Multiple Choice Questions

1.(c)	2.(b)	3.(c)	4.(a)	5.(b)	6.(b)	7.(c)
8.(a)	9.(a)	10.(b)	11.(c)	12.(c)	13.(c)	14.(c)
15.(d)	16.(c)	17.(d)	18.(b)	19.(a)	20.(b)	21.(a)
22.(c)	23.(b)	24.(c)	25.(d)	26.(c)	27.(a)	28.(a)
29.(d)	30.(d)	31.(a)	32.(c)	33.(d)	34.(a)	35.(b)
36.(c)	37.(a)	38.(d)	39.(d)	40.(d)	41.(b)	42.(b)
43.(b)	44.(a)	45.(c)	46.(d)	47.(a)	48.(c)	49.(c)
50.(c)	51.(d)	52.(c)	53.(d)	54.(a)	55.(a)	56.(b)
57.(a)	58.(b)	59.(d)	60.(d)	61.(a)	62.(d)	63.(d)
64.(a)	65.(c)	66.(a)	67.(a)	68.(d)	69.(c)	70.(b)
71.(b)	72.(d)	73.(b)	74.(a)	75.(a)	76.(d)	77.(a)
78.(d)	79.(d)	80.(c)	81.(c)	82.(c)	83.(a)	84.(b)
85.(c)	86.(d)	87.(d)	88.(a)	89.(a)	90.(a)	91.(a)
92.(b)	93.(a)	94.(d)	95.(b)	96.(d)	97.(a)	98.(d)
99.(d)	100.(a)					

Fill in the Blanks

1. 0.13-0.15 per cent
2. 0.17 per cent
3. Standard Plate Count (SPC)
4. Direct Microscopic Count (DMC)
5. Five lac
6. Leptospira
7. 1-5 lac
8. Somatic cell
9. Metylene blue and Resazurin
10. Dehydrogenase
11. Bacteria, leucocytes
12. More than 4 hr
13. 30,000CFU/ml
14. Phosphatase test
15. Alkaline Phosphatase
16. Disodium p-nitrophenyl phosphate
17. Milk and Milk Product Order

18. Spoilage organism, Pathogenic organism
19. Thermophilic, Mesophilic, Psychrophilic
20. Unsaturated
21. *Streptococcus lactis* var. *multigens*
22. *Bacillus circulans*
23. Rancid flavor
24. Sweet curdling
25. Rennin
26. *Alkaligens viscolactis*
27. Feed, fodder
28. More
29. 72 h
30. I131
31. Antibiotic residues or Bacteriophages
32. *Streptococcus agalactiae*
33. Bovine somatotrophin
34. Thermophilic
35. 25-30°C
36. 10 per cent
37. *Bacillus cereus*
38. Thermoduric
39. 4-5 hrs
40. 6.6-6.8
41. Sulfhydryl
42. Lipolytic bacteria
43. Soxlet
44. *Coxiella burnetti*
45. Batch holder method
46. 7days
47. Flow diversion valve
48. Regenration section
49. 137-150 °C, 1-2 sec
50. Bactofugation
51. Vacreation
52. Uperization
53. One month
54. *Bacillus subtilis*
55. *Bacillus stearothermophilus*
56. Maillard reaction
57. Lysine
58. Spore count
59. Turbidity test
60. 7 days
61. 60°C
62. 2 meter
63. 112mg/L
64. 42-52 cm
65. Central/State pollution control Board
66. Chlorine compound
67. 800
68. H_2O_2
69. p - dimethylaminobenzaldehyde
70. Rosailic acid
71. Iodine test
72. Fat
73. Increase
74. Baird Parker

75. Violet Red Bile Agar
76. *Listeria*
77. Dorset egg medium, Dubos medium
78. Allergic reaction
79. Trematol
80. Rat bite fever
81. *Listeria, Yersinea*
82. *Bacillus cereus*
83. Heat labile
84. Q fever
85. Tick borne encephalitis
86. *Cl. perfringens*
87. Leptospirosis
88. Udder
89. Milk ring test
90. Enteropathogenic *E. coli*
91. *Streptococci pyogenes*
92. Infected handlers, contaminated water
93. Liver
94. Contaminated water, carrier milkers
95. Lactoperoxidase
96. Thiocynate, H_2O_2
97. Substrate, Promoter
98. 60-80° C
99. *Bacillus stearothermophilus var.calidolactis*
100. Lipopolysaccharide.

MARK TRUE/FALSE

1. False
2. False
3. False
4. False
5. False
6. False
7. False
8. True
9. False
10. True
11. False
12. False
13. True
14. False
15. True
16. True
17. True
18. False
19. False
20. False
21. True
22. True
23. True
24. False
25. True
26. False
27. False
28. False
29. False
30. False
31. False
32. True
33. False
34. False
35. True
36. False
37. True
38. False
39. False
40. True
41. False
42. False
43. True
44. False
45. False
46. False
47. True
48. True
49. True
50. False
51. False
52. True
53. True
54. True
55. False
56. False
57. True
58. True
59. True
60. True

61. True	71. True	81. True	91. True
62. False	72. False	82. True	92. False
63. True	73. True	83. True	93. False
64. True	74. False	84. True	94. True
65. True	75. False	85. True	95. True
66. False	76. True	86. True	96. True
67. True	77. False	87. False	97. True
68. False	78. False	88. False	98. False
69. True	79. True	89. False	99. True
70. True	80. True	90. True	100. True

Matching Type Questions

Part A

1.	J	6.	A
2.	I	7.	E
3.	H	8.	C
4.	G	9.	D
5.	F	10.	B

Part B

1.	F	6.	E
2.	G	7.	J
3.	B	8.	I
4.	A	9.	C
5.	H	10.	D

Part C

1.	J	6.	B
2.	I	7.	E
3.	G	8.	H
4.	A	9.	D
5.	F	10.	C

Part D

1.	C	6.	K
2.	D	7.	J
3.	E	8.	F
4.	B	9.	G
5.	A	10.	I

Part E

1.	F	6.	B
2.	E	7.	A
3.	G	8.	D
4.	H	9.	I
5.	C	10.	J

Part F

1.	F	6.	A
2.	G	7.	B
3.	H	8.	C
4.	I	9.	D
5.	J	10.	E

Chapter 3
Meat Hygiene

MULTIPLE CHOICE QUESTIONS

1. **Splashing is frequently seen in______ stunning method:**

   (a) Gaseous (b) Electrical

   (c) Mechanical (d) Percussive

2. **The intensity of light at inspection site should be:**

   (a) 500 LUX (b) 220 LUX

   (c) 540 LUX (d) 100LUX

3. **The temperature of meat cutting room must not exceed:**

   (a) 12°C (b) 22°C

   (c) 4°C (d) 37°C

4. **The offal which is a rich source of vitamin A is:**

   (a) Spleen (b) Liver

   (c) Tongue (d) Kidney

5. **A female sheep which has not yet borne a lamb is called:**

   (a) Gimmer (b) Ewe

   (c) Cast ewe (d) Wether

6. **Spleen is not included in pluck in:**
   (a) Sheep (b) Goat
   (c) Pig (d) Cattle

7. **Following are known as meat lymph nodes in pig:**
   (a) Prefemoral and popliteal (b) Prefemoral and prescapular
   (c) Axillary and popliteal (d) Ischiatic and popliteal

8. **The lymph nodes are numerous and present in grape like cluster in:**
   (a) Dog (b) Cattle
   (c) Horse (d) Sheep

9. **Slaughter of _______ is a social and religious taboo among Buddhist:**
   (a) Cow (b) Pig
   (c) Yak (d) Deer

10. **The most important intrinsic factor that affects microbial spoilage is:**
    (a) Temperature (b) Water activity
    (c) pH (d) Relative humidity

11. **The intensity of light in meat plant at routine work area should be:**
    (a) 20 Foot candle (b) 50 Foot candle
    (c) 40 Foot candle (d) 60 Foot candle

12. **Almost black colored blood with sweet and repulsive odour is characteristic in :**
    (a) Dog (b) Cattle
    (c) Horse (d) Sheep

13. **The strength of chlorine for sanitation of meat plant should range between:**
    (a) 130-250ppm (b) 50-100ppm
    (c) 50-150ppm (d) 250-350ppm

14. An emergency slaughter hall have the lairage facility for at least:

(a) 4 animals (b) 15 animals

(b) 10 animals (d) 20 animals

15. Free bullet pistol is most suitable for stunning of:

(a) Horse (b) Pig

(c) Cattle (d) Sheep

16. Percentage of bone in Bobby Calf is :

(a) 25 per cent (b) 50 per cent

(c) 75 per cent (d) 85 per cent

17. The height of dressing rail for cattle should be :

(a) 3.5 meter (b) 3.0 meter

(c) 2.5 meter (d) 2.0 meter

18. The height of dressing rail for small animal should be:

(a) 2.5 m (b) 3.5 m

(c) 3.0 m (d) 4.0 m

19. The height of bleeding rail for large animal should be:

(a) 3.5 m (b) 3.0

(c) 4.5 m (d) 4.0 m

20. The height of bleeding rail for small animal should be:

(a) 3.5 m (b) 3.0

(c) 4.5 m (d) 4.0 m

21. The strength of electrical current recommended for pigs is:

(a) 250V, 10 sec (b) 75V, 10 sec

(c) 150V, 5sec (d) 70V,15sec

22. The pistol muzzle should be placed about________above the level of eye in pig in captive bolt stunning method:

(a) 1.5cm (b) 2.5cm

(c) 3.5cm (d) 4.5cm

23. Which one aspect of ante-mortem inspection requires the Veterinarian to identify Notifiable disease?

(a) Public health (b) Animal welfares

(c) Animal health (d) None of above

24. The carcass yield of calf is:

(a) 50.0 per cent (b) 35.0 per cent

(c) 70.0 per cent (d) 63.0 per cent

25. The component of a modern abattoir where animals are allowed to rest before slaughter is called:

(a) Mini abattoir (b) Detained meat room

(c) Lairage (d) Isolation box

26. Which of the following step is performed in last during post-mortem examination?

(a) Cervical inspection (b) Carcase inspection

(c) Visceral inspection (d) Lymph node inspection.

27. The conditions in which rigor mortis may be absent, is/are:

(a) Fever (b) Exhausted

(c) Fatigue (d) All of above

28. The molecular technique where restriction enzymes are used for meat speciation is:

(a) IEF (b) RFLP

(c) RAPD, (d) SDS-PAGE.

29. The species that have largest length of muscle fibre is:

(a) Cattle (b) Pig

(c) Horse (d) Goat

30. Heparin is obtained from________part of animal:

(a) Stomach (b) Blood

(c) Small intestine (d) Bone

31. The following by products are obtained from intestine except:

(a) Heparin (b) Casing

(c) Insulin (d) Surgical suture

32. Gelatin is an animal by product obtained from:

(a) Bone (b) Hide and skin

(c) Intestine (d) Blood

33. The meat affected with cyst of *Taenia solium* is called:

(a) Measly beef (b) Both of abovek

(c) Measly pork (d) None of above

34. The smallest meat borne tapeworm, which is composed of a head and three segment:

(a) *Taenia solium* (b) *Taenia saginata*

(c) *Taenia* (d) *Echinococcus granulosus*

35. The biochemical technique where isoelectric point is used for meat speciation is:

(a) IEF (b) RFLP

(c) RAPD (d) SDS-PAGE

36. The species that have largest number of lymph node is:

(b) Cattle (b) Pig

(c) Horse (d) Goat

37. Bone taint is a deep seated spoilage of meat caused by:

(a) *Clostridium sporogenes* (b) *Clostridium putrifaciens*

(c) *Clostridium purtificum* (d) All of the above

38. Phosphorescence in frozen meat is caused by:

(a) *Pseudomonas aerugenosa* (b) Pseudomonas synxantha

(c) *Pseudomonas fluorescence* (d) None of the above

39. All the following are sarcoplasmic proteins found in meat except:

(a) Myoglobin (b) Heamoglobin

(c) Troponin (d) Glycolytic enzymes

40. Inspection of carcass after evisceration is also called:

(a) Cervical inspection (b) Visceral inspection

(c) Rail inspection (d) Post mortem

41. Transit fever is a condition that chiefly affects :

(a) Cattle (b) Poultry

(c) Pig (d) Horse

42. Chances of back bleeding are more in :

(a) Cattle (b) Poultry

(c) Pig (d) Horse

43. Brain cannot be used for edible purpose in :

(a) Percussive stunning (b) Gaseous stunning

(c) Invasive type stunning (d) Electrical stunning

44. Causes of shrink in live weight after transportation are greater due to :

(a) Fasting and improper watering (b) Excretion of waste

(c) Sweating and exhaustion (d) Both (a) and (b)

45. In addition to larynx, trachea, liver, lung and heart, pluck in case of sheep also includes:

(a) Spleen (b) Oesophagus

(c) Kidney (d) Omasum

46. The chemical used to inhibit the growth of *Clostridium botulinum* in meat is:

(a) Nitrite (b) Sorbate

(c) Benzoate (d) Lactate

47. The water requirement of an abattoir for cattle may be calculated at the rate of:

(a) 400-600lt/cattle (b) 250-400lt/cattle

(c) 700-1000lt/cattle (d) None of these

48. The water requirement for sheep and goat abattoir may be calculated at the rate of:

(a) 400-600lt/head (b) 250-400lt/head

(c) 700-1000lt/head (d) None of these

49. Determination of adulteration in meat by SDS-PAGE is based on:

(a) Iso- electric point (b) DNA hybridization

(c) Molecular wt. of protein (d) Ag-Ab reaction

50. Color of mesenteric lymph node in cattle is:

(a) Grey (b) Red

(c) Black (d) White

51. Fatal syncope or Hertzod is a synonym of:

(a) PSE (b) PSS

(c) DFD (d) BSE

52. The most suitable method for disposal of carcass affected with highly infectious diseases is:

(a) Burial (b) Incineration

(c) Wet rendering (d) Dry rendering

53. The final moisture concentration of meat preserved by drying should be:

(a) 4 per cent (b) 15 per cent

(c) 10 per cent (d) 20 per cent

54. In modern slaughter house, the temperature of cutting room must not exceed:

(a) 5°C (b) 12°C

(c) 20°C (d) 25°C

55. In chilling room, the temperature of carcass should be reduced to:

(a) 3°C (b) 15°C

(c) 7°C (d) 0°C

56. The most appropriate measure to determine the concentration of abattoir waste is:

(a) BOD (b) COD

(c) Total solid (d) dry matter

57. The cow slaughter is strictly banned in the State of:

(a) Delhi (b) Kerala

(c) Assam (d) West Bengal

58. The method of disposal used for unsound meat or offals obtained from the animals died of non- contagious disease is:

(a) Burial (b) Rendering

(c) Incineration (d) Burning

59. The slaughter may be delayed in the condition of :

(a) Excessively fatigued (b) Under treatment

(c) Excitement (d) All of above

60. The term giblet is used to denote the______ organs:

(a) Stomach, intestine

(b) Tongue, oesophagus, trachea

(c) Heart, liver, lung

(d) Heart, liver and gizzard

61. The intrinsic factor that causes delay in the onset of rigor mortis is:

(a) Highly active Muscle (b) High level of ATP

(c) High Env. temperature (d) Highly active species

62. The halothane sensitive gene is found in ______ breed/s of pig:

(a) Landrace (b) Poland china

(c) Pietrain (d) All of above

63. The major end product of anaerobic glycolysis in muscle is:

(a) Lactic acid (b) ATP

(c) CO_2 (d) Pyruvate

64. Kidney fat is abundant in (animal species):

(a) Sheep (b) Cattle

(c) Goat (d) Pig

65. Amonical odour is the characteristic of :

(a) Pork (b) Mutton

(c) Chevon (d) Beef

66. A thick subcutaneous fatty layer is a characteristic of:

(a) Pork (b) Mutton

(c) Chevon (d) Beef

67. Unhygienic and unauthorized killing of food animal is known as:

(a) Ritual slaughter (b) Clandestine slaughter

(c) Human slaughter (d) Sacrifice

68. An animal showing excessive laceration may be placed in the category of:

(a) Emergency slaughter

(b) Slaughter under special condition

(c) Delayed slaughter

(d) Casualty slaughter

69. An incision to be given without any pause, pressure, tearing, stabbing, slanting is the thumb rule of:

(a) Halal method (b) Clandestine slaughter

(c) Humane Method (d) Jewish method

70. Lymph nodes are absent in:

(a) Poultry (b) Pig

(c) Horse (d) Cattle

71. 'Warmed-over flavour' in meat is caused by:

(a) Volatile compound (b) Steroid

(c) Phospholipase (d) H_2O_2

72. An imaginary zone around the animal, which it always tries to maintain by moving away while being handled is called:

(a) Fight zone (b) Flight zone

(c) Fright zone (d) Prohibited zone

73. The condition seen in tetanus affected animal on antemortem inspection is:

(a) Locked jaw (b) Dropped jaw

(c) Lumpy Jaw (d) Open jaw

74. The organ of choice for determination of antibiotic residues in meat is:

(a) Liver (b) Kidney

(c) Both (a) and (b) (d) Spleen

75. The change that is not associated with incomplete bleeding is:

(a) Blood in left ventricle (b) Engorged S/C blood vessel

(c) Dark flabby flesh (d) Cloudy swelling

76. The test used for detection of icterus in meat is:

(a) Rimmington and Fowrie test (b) Rothera's test

(c) Melachite green test (d) Casoni test

77. Boiling test in meat should be performed for detection of:

(a) Abnormal odour (b) Freshness

(c) Abnormal taste (d) Staleness

78. The condition not found in an emaciated animal is:

(a) Wrinkled and dry skin (b) Prominent bones

(c) Rough hair coat (d) Prominent eyes

79. The change not associated with porcine stress syndrome is:

(a) Decrease in temperature (b) Arrhythmia

(c) Skin blanching (d) Dyspnoea

80. As per ICMSF standards, the count of Salmonella in good quality meat should be:

(a) 0 (b) Not more than 1/g

(c) 1/10g (d) 10/10 g

81. The color of colonies of *Staphylococci* on Baird Parker medium is:

(a) Yellow (b) Jet Black

(c) Violet (d) Pink

82. The color of colonies of *Salmonella* on Brilliant green agar medium is:

(a) Pale Yellow (b) Green

(c) Violet (d) Pink

83. Spleen is congested and contains tiny foci of necrosis in bovine salmonellosis. This spleenomegaly is known as:

(a) Burst spleen (b) Board spleen

(c) Slaughter spleen (d) Balloon spleen

84. The extract release volume of good quality meat should be:

(a) More than 30 ml (b) More than 20ml

(c) More than 25ml (d) less than 20 ml

85. The device used for gaseous stunning is known as:

(a) Oval tunnel (b) Ferris wheel

(c) Dip lift (d) All of above

86. The method of gaseous stunning, having largest thorough put is:

(a) Oval tunnel (b) Ferris wheel

(c) Dip lift (d) pilot wheel

87. On ante mortem inspection, if uncontrolled haemorrahages are seen, the judgment should be:

(a) Casualty slaughter (b) Delayed slaughter

(c) Emergency slaughter (d) Unfit for slaughter

88. The judgement of emergency slaughter is given in case of:

(a) Postpartum paraplegia (b) Uterine prolapse

(c) Lactation tetany (d) Recumbency

89. The animal should be declared 'unfit for slaughter' after antemortem examination if it is suffering from:

(a) Rabies (b) Haemorrhagic septicemia

(c) Tetanus (d) All of above

90. If the animal stock is found very dirty on ante mortem inspection, the judgement should be:

(a) Casualty slaughter (b) Slaughter at last

(c) Delayed slaughter (d) Unfit for slaughter

91. The term 'bob-veal' is used to denote the meat of:

(a) Day old calf (b) 10 days old calf

(c) 7 days old calf (d) 30 days old calf

92. The major by-product obtained from animal fat is/are:

(a) Candy (b) Soap and detergent

(c) Chewingum (d) All of above

93. The possible source of contamination to establish critical control points in fresh meat production in buffalo abattoir is/are:

(a) Evisceration (b) Cutting

(c) Chilling (d) All of above

94. The humane method of slaughter by designing of a gaseous chamber to induce anaesthesia in animal to kill them, was developed for the first time by:

(a) Benjamin Ward Richordson (b) James Steel

(c) Martin Kaplan (d) John Snow

95. The blue print of slaughter house was developed by:

(a) Benjamin Ward Richardson (b) James Steel

(c) Martin Kaplan (d) John Snow

96. The main purpose of stunning is:

(a) To induce unconsciousness

(b) To improve meat quality

(c) To enhance bleeding efficiency

(d) To relieve pain to animal

97. The person who assist the cutter in Jewish method is called:

(a) Schochet (b) Kosher

(c) Shomer (d) Chalef

98. Trimethylamine level more than 7 mg per cent in fish meat indicates:

(a) Fresh fish (b) Onset of spoilage

(c) Spoiled fish (d) Very fresh

99. The first bacterium to invade the carcass from bowel after death is:

(a) *E. coli* (b) *Klebsiella*

(c) *Cl. perfringens* (d) *Pseudomonas*

100. Use of antibiotics should be withheld atleat _______ prior to slaughter:

(a) 3 days (b) 5 days

(c) 15 days (d) 20 days

FILL IN THE BLANKS

1. Toughness in muscle after the onset of rigor mortis is caused by_______.
2. A knife is inserted in _______ space to severe medulla oblongata in 'evernazione method'.
3. Transit tetany occurs in cows in _______ (stage) during long journey.
4. Processing of unfit meat and offal into useful product is called _______.
5. Intramuscular deposition of fat is called_______.
6. Loss of weight during transport is called _______.
7. BSE is transmitted to man by ingestion of _______.
8. Dark, firm and dry meat is more common in _______.
9. Accumulation of firm, fibrous protein substance in body tissue is called _______.
10. Greenish discoloration of crop and cloaca with putrid smell is called_______.

11. The person who perfoms acts of slaughter in 'Jewish method' is called _______.

12. Dark red to bluish color and sweet and repulsive odour are the characteristics of_______ flesh.

13. 'Canpak system' is an example of _______ dressing system.

14. The iodine value of unsaturated fatty acid is highest in_______.

15. Blackish discoloration of bronchial lymph node is indication of _______.

16. Superficial congestion of skin results in gaseous anaesthesia if period of CO_2 exposure is _______.

17. The height of overhead bleeding rail should be _______ above the floor.

18. Pale, soft, exudative condition is more commonly seen in _______ (animal species).

19. Country in which pork is the meat of choice is _______.

20. Pithing rod greater than 60 cm may destroy the _______ nerve resulting in slaughter spleen condition.

21. The animal species that have innate tendency to follow one another is _______.

22. The speed of vehicle carrying the animals should not exceed _______.

23. Head of animal is drawn towards _______ in 'Halal method'.

24. Feeding in lairage is required only when detention time is longer than _______.

25. Barking is a pathological condition caused by high scalding temperature in _______.

26. Necrosis of brisket fat in cattle and sheep is called_______.

27. The knife used in 'evernazione method' is called _______.

28. Removal of blood vessels from hind quarter in 'Jewish method' is called _______.

29. The skin of pig should be examined for presence of lesions of _______ on post mortem examination.

30. The escape of watery blood stained fluid from frozen meat after thawing is called _______.
31. Accumulation of fluid in musculature is called _______.
32. The organ where the onset of rigor mortis is seen within an hour of slaughter is _______.
33. Nitrite in curing mixture plays an important role in _______.
34. In pig, bleeding is achieved by severing_______.
35. Highest dressing percentage is met in_______ (animal species).
36. Passage of electrical current in stunning is enhanced by_______.
37. Per capita availability of meat in India is_______per annum.
38. The best method of stunning in case of large animal is_______.
39. Udder is included in carcase in _______ (animal species).
40. Dressing percentage in cattle is_______.
41. Horse meat is preferred in _______country.
42. Antioxidant property of smoke is due to _______.
43. Bleeding should take place within_______ after leaving the gas chamber.
44. The technique of sealing of rectum is known as _______.
45. ' Jewish method' of slaughter is known as _______.
46. Technical term for deer meat is _______.
47. Body of Jewish law is known as _______.
48. The burning of hair stump is known as _______.
49. The ultimate effect of general adaptation syndrome is_______ in blood glucose and ketone.
50. PSE is also known as _______.
51. Eating of dog flesh is known as _______.
52. Neck-stab method of slaughter is also known as_______
53. The number of modern export oriented abattoirs in India is _______.

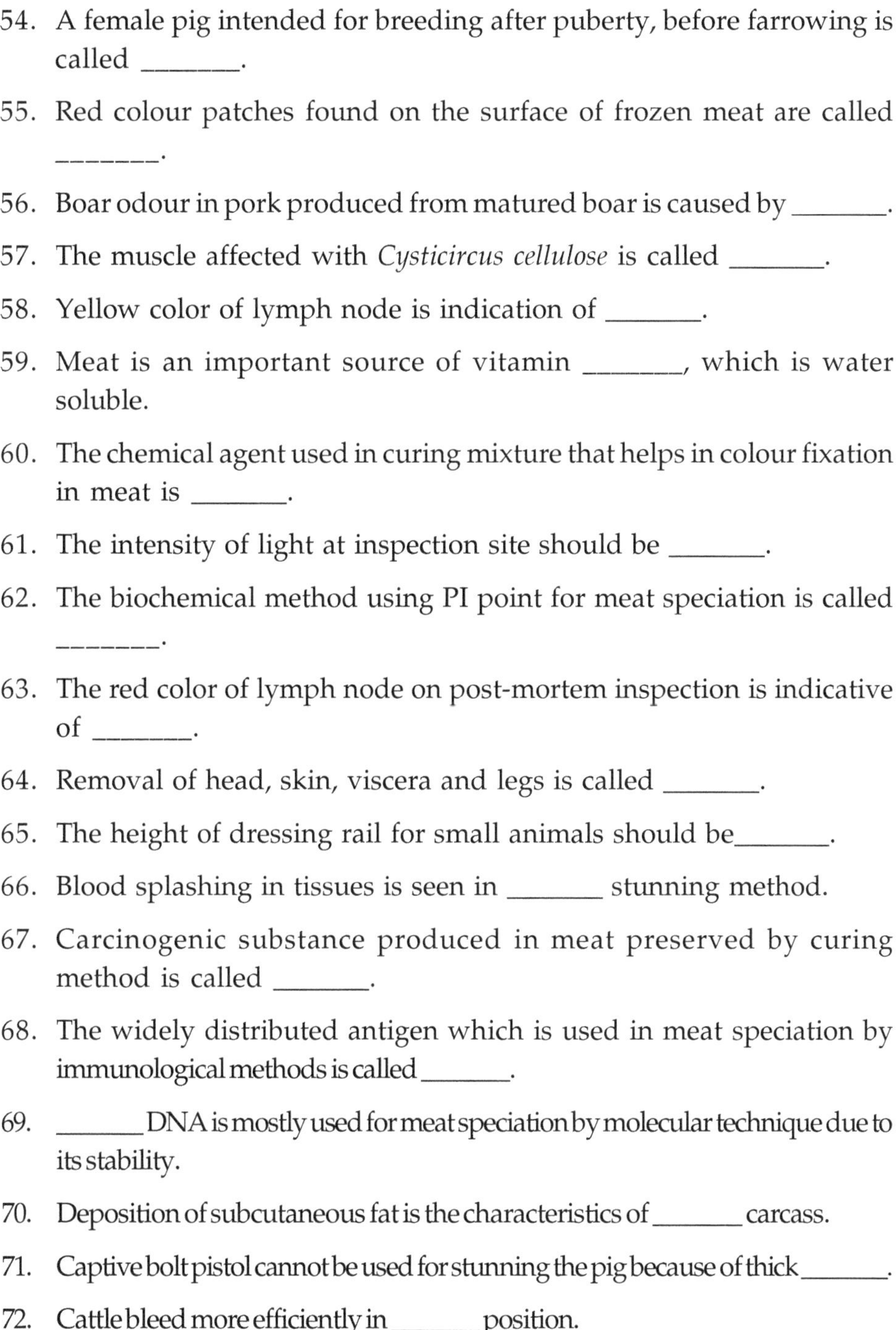

54. A female pig intended for breeding after puberty, before farrowing is called _______.
55. Red colour patches found on the surface of frozen meat are called _______.
56. Boar odour in pork produced from matured boar is caused by _______.
57. The muscle affected with *Cysticircus cellulose* is called _______.
58. Yellow color of lymph node is indication of _______.
59. Meat is an important source of vitamin _______, which is water soluble.
60. The chemical agent used in curing mixture that helps in colour fixation in meat is _______.
61. The intensity of light at inspection site should be _______.
62. The biochemical method using PI point for meat speciation is called _______.
63. The red color of lymph node on post-mortem inspection is indicative of _______.
64. Removal of head, skin, viscera and legs is called _______.
65. The height of dressing rail for small animals should be_______.
66. Blood splashing in tissues is seen in _______ stunning method.
67. Carcinogenic substance produced in meat preserved by curing method is called _______.
68. The widely distributed antigen which is used in meat speciation by immunological methods is called_______.
69. _______DNA is mostly used for meat speciation by molecular technique due to its stability.
70. Deposition of subcutaneous fat is the characteristics of_______carcass.
71. Captive bolt pistol cannot be used for stunning the pig because of thick_______.
72. Cattle bleed more efficiently in_______position.

73. Meat of calves, exclusively fed on milk and slaughtered at the age of 2-4 month after attaining 70 kg weight, is called ______.

74. Meat of calves exclusively fed on barley diet and slaughtered at the age of 4 month after attaining 90 kg weight is called ______.

75. Transit fever is also known as ______ fever.

76. In case of lean carcass, water to protein ratio is ______ than 4:1.

77. Exposure of meat to low temperature immediately after slaughter may cause upto ______ cold shortening.

78. The CO_2 concentration in air for stunning of poultry should be ______for______(time).

79. Bleeding in pig is performed by giving incision in a depression in front of ______by severing carotid artery and jugular vein.

80. An imaginary zone around the animal, which it endeavors to maintain by moving away when handlers enter into this zone, is called______.

81. A trained sheep accustomed to pass through lairage leading others is called ______.

82. In healthy animal, rigor mortis commences after______hours of slaughter.

83. The internal organs comprising larynx, trachea, liver, lung, heart which are removed together in dressing are called______.

84. The internal organs comprising larynx, trachea, lungs, heart and liver constitute pluck in______and______(animal species).

85. In pigs______remains attached to the trachea, that is why it is included in pluck.

86. The term used by Jews for meat which is unfit for human consumption is ______.

87. The deep seated spoilage of carcass by anaerobic bacteria where level of fat is fairly high is called______.

88. The glandular structure that must be examined during postmortem inspection is called______.

89. Warmed over flavour in cured meat is build up due to______

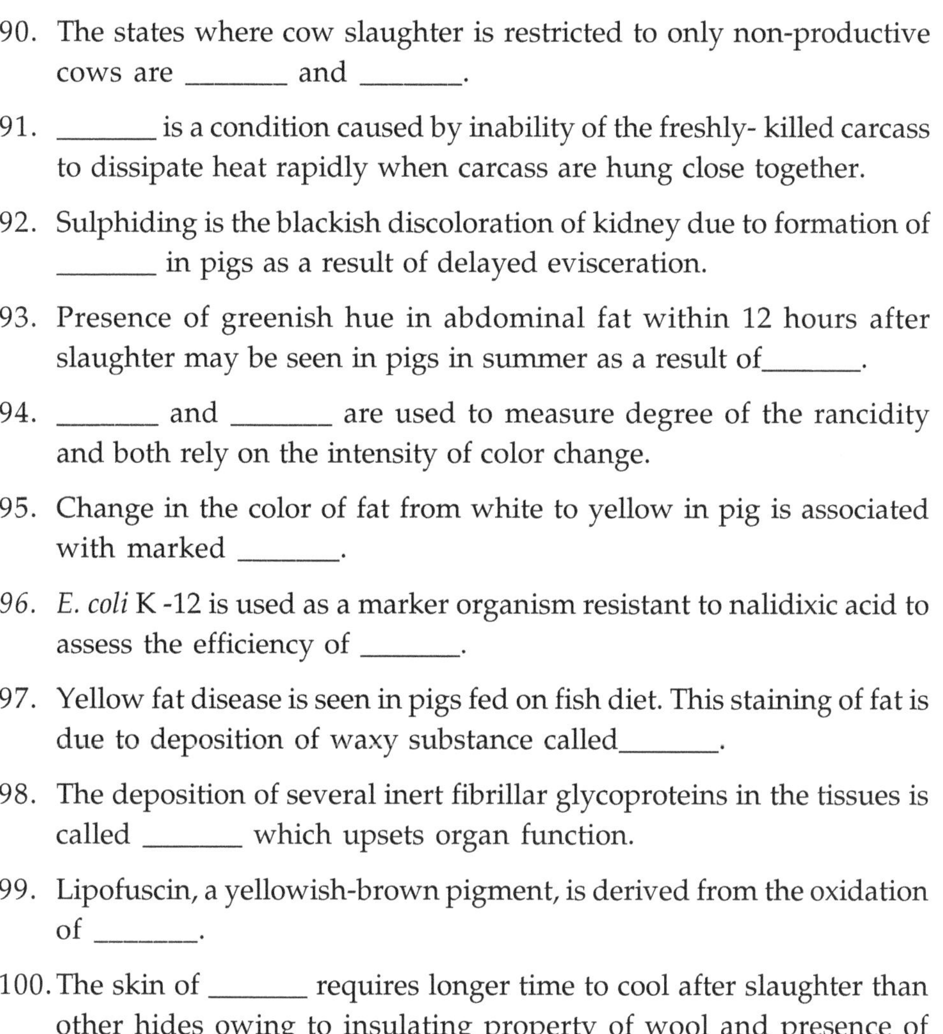

90. The states where cow slaughter is restricted to only non-productive cows are _______ and _______.

91. _______ is a condition caused by inability of the freshly- killed carcass to dissipate heat rapidly when carcass are hung close together.

92. Sulphiding is the blackish discoloration of kidney due to formation of _______ in pigs as a result of delayed evisceration.

93. Presence of greenish hue in abdominal fat within 12 hours after slaughter may be seen in pigs in summer as a result of_______.

94. _______ and _______ are used to measure degree of the rancidity and both rely on the intensity of color change.

95. Change in the color of fat from white to yellow in pig is associated with marked _______.

96. *E. coli* K -12 is used as a marker organism resistant to nalidixic acid to assess the efficiency of _______.

97. Yellow fat disease is seen in pigs fed on fish diet. This staining of fat is due to deposition of waxy substance called_______.

98. The deposition of several inert fibrillar glycoproteins in the tissues is called _______ which upsets organ function.

99. Lipofuscin, a yellowish-brown pigment, is derived from the oxidation of _______.

100. The skin of _______ requires longer time to cool after slaughter than other hides owing to insulating property of wool and presence of grease.

MARK TRUE/FALSE

1. DFD meat is perfectly fit for consumption.
2. Animal behavior is not very important consideration in lairage design.
3. Most of the meat exported from India belongs to goat.
4. Refractive index of eye fluid is used as indicator to determine the freshness of fish.
5. Removal of large blood vessels in 'Jewish method' is called exsanguinations.
6. Rigor mortis goes undetected in febrile or fatigued animals.
7. High redox potential in meat favors the growth of anaerobic bacteria.
8. Pigs are more susceptible than cattle to strident voice in lairage.
9. Eating of swine, dead animal and blood is forbidden in Muslim community.
10. Examination of adhesion in thoracic cavity is called searching in 'Jewish method'.
11. Food and water must be offered to animal at every 6 hours interval during journey period.
12. The meat produced from exhausted animal will have high pH.
13. The knife used to kill animals in 'Jewish method' is called 'Puntilla'.
14. Bobby calves are usually slaughtered at the age of 7 week.
15. Horse meat is common on dinner table in many European countries.
16. An emaciated animal can be passed for slaughter.
17. Buffalo meat is lean and contains less cholesterol than cattle.
18. Head and kidneys are excluded from carcass yield in case of pig.
19. Pigs prefer to move as a group, with their comrades on either side.
20. Water holding capacity of muscle decreases after the onset of rigor mortis.

21. Fiber optic probes are more accurate than pH meter in detection of PSE and DFD condition in meat.
22. The maximum slope of loading or unloading ramp should be 45°.
23. Holding of cattle in lairage should be restricted to 4 hours to maximize carcass yield and meat quality.
24. Horizontal scalding tank is better than vertical tank as it reduces the incidence of PSE.
25. Scalding and singing are major source of contamination in pig abattoir.
26. Botulism is an important meat borne disease transmitted by low acid canned food having type A and B toxins of *Clostridium botulinum.*
27. The CO_2 concentration in air for stunning of poultry should be 90 per cent.
28. Quality of meat produced by gaseous stunning is better than electrical stunning.
29. Bluish discoloration of skin in gaseous stunning is due to high concentration of CO_2.
30. The *E. coli* count in good quality meat should be 10/g in 3 samples and 100/g in 2 samples as per ICMSF.
31. Wax stripping is done in ducks to facilitate de-feathering.
32. Rest interval during journey should not exceed 12h for sheep, goat, pig and cattle.
33. Characteristic fall in the pH of meat from 7.0 to 5.5 takes place in 24-48 hours of slaughter in cattle.
34. Head to back/leg electrical stunning produces lower incidence of blood splashing.
35. Both casuality slaughter and emergency slaughter are done in emergency slaughter hall.
36. In case of poorness, water to protein ratio is greater than 4:1.
37. A carcass showing 'anasarca' on postmortem inspection should be totally rejected.

38. An icteric carcass can be passed for human consumption, if jaundice disappears after chilling.
39. Bunging is done in cattle to prevent contamination from gastrointestinal tract.
40. Slaughter spleen, a condition showing enlargement of spleen is caused by faulty sticking.
41. Horse fat contains about 1-2 per cent linolenic acid, while in other species it is less than 0.1 per cent.
42. The diameter and depth of air sac decreases with the aging of egg.
43. Blood yield is more in bulls than cows.
44. Sheep and goat can be mixed together while transportation.
45. Trichinellosis is classical example of meat borne disease.
46. Carcass yield is expressed as per cent of dead wt. of animal.
47. Bleeding in swine is achieved by severing anterior venacava and Bracheocephalic trunk.
48. Stunning is strictly forbidden in 'Halal' method of slaughter.
49. Plenty of water while rest reduces the microbial load in intestine.
50. Bleeding is more efficient in electrical stunning as compared to gaseous stunning.
51. The mesenteric lymph nodes of ox are almost white in colour.
52. Preservation of meat by ionizing radiations at the dose level > 1 mega RAD is called radurisaion.
53. Half of all breeds of goat are found in Asian subcontinent.
54. In an infection, the lymph nodes are enlarged, while in starved animal, involution particularly of mesenteric lymph node may occur.
55. Dehiding is followed by bleeding in line method.
56. A lean carcass may be approved as fit for human consumption.
57. Domestic yak is considered to have descended from wild yak *i.e., Bos taurus.*
58. Rabbit meat is high in protein but low in fat and cholesterol.
59. Exposure of meat to low temperature immediately after slaughter results in excessive shortening of muscle, which is known as 'thaw rigor'.

60. The loss of live weight during journey is greater than that which is solely caused by fasting for a similar period.
61. An animal suffering with tetanus can be passed for slaughter for human consumption.
62. Captive bolt pistol cannot be used for stunning the pig.
63. Bleeding in pig is achieved by severing carotid artery and jugular vein.
64. Redurized meat can be kept safely at room temperature for long time.
65. 'Allanasons Limited' is the largest meat processing enterprise in India.
66. Cold shortening may reach upto 50 per cent due to exposure of meat to low temperature immediately after slaughter.
67. The imperfectly bled animal may show blood in right ventricle.
68. Drip losses are more in blast freezing than slow freezing method of preservation.
69. Mithun is larger than gaur and smaller than domestic cattle.
70. Spleen is not included in pluck in pig.
71. Feeding and watering before slaughter is allowed in 'Halal method'.
72. The temperature of water should be 82°C for cleaning greasy surfaces.
73. Yellow color of lymph node is indicative of icterus.
74. Rigor mortis is either absent or transient in fevered carcase.
75. Flaying is replaced by scalding in pig.
76. Chevon is darker in colour than mutton.
77. Glycogen content is highest in buffalo meat.
78. Mithun is developed by crossing Indian bison and domestic cattle.
79. Marbling is very much prominent in horse meat.
80. Halothane gene is found in pig.
81. Carcass yield in pig is defined as weight of two sides excluding head, blood, viscera.
82. Casting pen facility is provided in the slaughter hall to ensure humane tailling of animal.

83. 'Tripery' is a room for storage of hide and skin.
84. Stunning is not strictly prohibited in 'Jewish method'.
85. Marbling is usually absent in goat but prominent in bullock meat.
86. Carcass yield is highest in bullocks.
87. Animal must face towards engine to prevent being frightened during journey.
88. Onset of rigor mortis is delayed in stressed animal due to low level of glycogen and ATP.
89. Small abattoir unit is capable of handling 10 cattle, 20sheep and10 pigs.
90. A detailed ante mortem examination can represent 50 per cent of meat inspection.
91. India ranks eighth in meat production and fifth in egg production in world.
92. High voltage electrical stunner works at 300V for 10 minutes.
93. An animal suffering from FMD can be declared fit for slaughter on ante mortem examination.
94. Pre-slaughter feeding of sugar improves meat quality.
95. The production of modern meat plant should be as high as 5000 cattle, 10,000 sheep, 3500 pigs every 10 hours.
96. Sheep bled in horizontal position lose approximately 10 per cent more blood than those suspended vertically.
97. Washing of livestock is contraindicated in temperate zone except in pigs.
98. Fresh meat intended for sale must be kept in chilling room and its temperature should not be more than 3° C.
99. Shrinkage during transportation is more in sheep than in cattle.
100. Sulphur stinkers are caused due to breakdown of sulphur containing proteins in high temperature processing by thermophilic *Clostridium nigrificance* and liberation of H_2S.

MATCHING TYPE QUESTIONS

Part A

Column – A		*Column – B*
1. Black spot	(__)	a. *Thamnidium*
2. Whiskers	(__)	b. *Sporotrichum*
3. Sulphur stinkers	(__)	c. Pseudomelanosis of kidney
4. Boar odour	(__)	d. *Clostridium nigrificans*
5. Watery pork	(__)	e. Unsaturated steroid
6. Sulphiding	(__)	f. *Cladosporium*
7. White spot	(__)	g. Stress
8. Blue green mould	(__)	h. *Clostridium sporogenes*
9. Phosphorescence	(__)	i. Penecillum
10. Bone taint	(__)	j. *Pseudomonas phosphorescence*

Part B

Column – A		*Column – B*
1. Fuchet reagent	(__)	a. Carcase setting
2. Melachite green test	(__)	b. Knife
3. Back bleeding	(__)	c. Slaughter spleen
4. Faulty pithing	(__)	d. Bruises
5. Rigor mortis	(__)	e. Bleeding efficiency
6. Bobby calf	(__)	f. Oversticking
7. Veal calf	(__)	g. 1-7 days old
8. Puntilla	(__)	h. 3-4 month old
9. Ratites	(__)	i. Poultry
10. Giblet	(__)	j. Flightless bird

Part C

Column – A		Column – B
1. Knackeries	(__)	a. Stunning box
2. Tanneries	(__)	b. Disposal of unsound meat
3. Tripery	(__)	c. Processing of skin and hide
4. Knocking pen	(__)	d. Gut emptying room
5. Detained meat room	(__)	e. Flaying
6. Exsanguination	(__)	f. Tenderization
7. Line method	(__)	g. Bleeding
8. Aging	(__)	h. Emergency slaughter hall
9. Cradle	(__)	i. Canpak system
10. Mini abattoir	(__)	j. Final inspection of retained carcase

Part D

Column – A		Column – B
1. Wear and tear pigment	(__)	a. *T. solium*
2. Xanthosis	(__)	b. *T. saginata*
3. Heated beef	(__)	c. Cow
4. Seedy belly	(__)	d. Lamb
5. Downer syndrome	(__)	e. Melanosis of brain
6. Black pith	(__)	f. Melanosis of Udder
7. Wet carcase syndrome	(__)	g. Angiotoma
8. Plum pudding liver	(__)	h. sour side
9. Measly Pork	(__)	i. Brown atrophy
10. Measly beef	(__)	j. Lipofuscins

Part E

Column – A		*Column – B*
1. DFD	(__)	a. Watery Pork
2. PSE	(__)	b. Sour side
3. Red offals	(__)	c. Abomasums of calf
4. Green offals	(__)	d. Intestine
5. Heated beef	(__)	e. Stomach, Intestine
6. Rennet	(__)	f. Liver, Heart, Kidney
7. Sausage casing	(__)	g. Pig
8. Halothane gen	(__)	h. Cattle
9. Kosher	(__)	i. Unfit meat
10. Terefa	(__)	j. Fit meat

Part F

Column – A		*Column – B*
1. Smoking	(__)	a. Internal corrosion
2. Curing	(__)	b. Imperfect canning
3. Fermentation	(__)	c. Cold air with pressure
4. Thermal sterilization	(__)	d. Irradiation
5. Cold sterilization	(__)	e. Canning
6. Rad-appertization	(__)	f. Pasteurization
7. Blast freezing	(__)	g. Nitrosamine
8. Hurdle technology	(__)	h. Benzapyrin
9. Nitrate swell	(__)	i. Lactic acid bacteria
10. Hydrogen swell	(__)	j. Combination of preservation technique

Part G:

Column – A		Column – B
1. Congenital phorhyria	(__)	a. Parturient paresis
2. Yellow fat disease	(__)	b. Q fever
3. Xanthosis	(__)	c. Shipping fever
4. Amyloidosis	(__)	d. Pink tooth
5. Dripping	(__)	e. Ceroid
6. Sodium chloride	(__)	f. Brown atrophy
7. Phosphates	(__)	g. Fibrinous protein in body tissue
8. Transit ferver	(__)	h. Weeping
9. Abattoir fever	(__)	i. reduces water activity
10. Downer syndrome	(__)	j. Increases water holding capacity

ANSWERS

Multiple Choice Qustions

1.(b)	2.(c)	3.(a)	4.(b)	5.(a)	6.(c)	7.(a)
8.(c)	9.(c)	10.(a)	11.(a)	12.(c)	13.(a)	14.(a)
15.(a)	16.(b)	17.(a)	18.(c)	19.(c)	20.(a)	21.(b)
22.(b)	23.(c)	24.(d)	25.(c)	26.(b)	27.(d)	28.(b)
29.(b)	30.(c)	31.(c)	32.(a)	33.(c)	34.(d)	35.(a)
36.(c)	37.(d)	38.(c)	39.(c)	40.(c)	41.(a)	42.(c)
43.(c)	44.(d)	45.(a)	46.(a)	47.(c)	48.(b)	49.(c)
50.(c)	51.(b)	52.(b)	53.(a)	54.(b)	55.(c)	56.(b)
57.(a)	58.(b)	59.(d)	60.(d)	61.(b)	62.(d)	63.(a)
64.(c)	65.(b)	66.(a)	67.(b)	68.(a)	69.(d)	70.(a)
71.(c)	72.(c)	73.(a)	74.(c)	75.(d)	76.(a)	77.(a)
78.(d)	79.(a)	80.(a)	81.(b)	82.(a)	83.(b)	84.(c)
85.(d)	86.(a)	87.(c)	88.(b)	89.(d)	90.(c)	91.(c)
92.(d)	93.(d)	94.(a)	95.(a)	96.(d)	97.(c)	98.(c)
99.(a)	100.(b)					

Fill in the Blanks

1. Actomyosine
2. Atlantooccipital space
3. Pregnancy
4. Rendering
5. Marbling
6. Shrinkage
7. Beef
8. Cattle
9. Amyloidosis
10. Green stuck
11. Schochet
12. Horse
13. Overhead rail system
14. Horse
15. Anthracosis
16. Long
17. 2.7 meter
18. Pig
19. China
20. Splanchnic Nerve

21. Sheep
22. 40 Km/h
23. Mecca
24. 24 hour
25. Poultry
26. Putty Brisket
27. Puntilla
28. Porging
29. Swine erysipelas
30. Dripping/weeping
31. Anasarca
32. Heart
33. Color fixation
34. Anterior venacava, bracheocephalic trunk
35. Pig/poultry
36. Water spray
37. 4.6/kg
38. Captive bolt
39. Heifer
40. 30-35 per cent
41. European
42. Phenol
43. 30 sec
44. Bunging
45. Schechita
46. Venesion
47. Talmud
48. Singing
49. Increase
50. Watery pork
51. Kinophagia
52. Evernazion
53. 13
54. Gilt
55. Freezer burn
56. Steroid
57. Measly pork
58. Fatty infiltration
59. B_{12}
60. Nitrate or Nitrite
61. 540 LUX
62. Iso-electrical focussing
63. Inefficient bleeding, congestion
64. Dressing
65. 2.5 m
66. Electrical
67. Nitrosamine
68. BE antigen
69. Mitochondrial
70. Pig
71. Frontal bone
72. Head down
73. Veal
74. Barley beef
75. Shipping
76. Less
77. 44 per cent
78. 73-77 per cent, 15 sec.
79. Sternum
80. Flight zone

81. Zudas sheep
82. 9-12
83. Pluck
84. Sheep, calf
85. Oesophagus
86. Terefa
87. Bone taint
88. Lymph node
89. Oxidative rancidity
90. Assam and West Bengal
91. Heated beef
92. Iron sulphide
93. Delayed evisceration
94. Kreis test and Thiobarbituric acid test
95. Rancidity
96. Dressing technique
97. Ceroid
98. Amyloidosis
99. Lipoproteins
100. Sheep.

MARK TRUE/FALSE

1. True
2. False
3. False
4. True
5. False
6. True
7. False
8. True
9. True
10. True
11. False
12. True
13. False
14. False
15. True
16. False
17. True
18. False
19. True
20. True
21. True
22. False
23. True
24. False
25. False
26. True
27. False
28. True
29. False
30. True
31. True
32. False
33. True
34. True
35. True
36. False
37. True
38. True
39. True
40. False
41. True
42. False
43. False
44. False
45. True
46. False
47. True
48. False
49. True
50. False
51. False
52. False
53. True
54. True
55. False
56. True
57. False
58. True
59. False
60. True
61. False
62. True
63. False
64. False
65. True
66. False
67. False
68. False
69. False
70. True
71. True
72. True

73. False	80. True	87. True	94. True
74. True	81. False	88. False	95. True
75. True	82. False	89. True	96. True
76. True	83. False	90. True	97. True
77. False	84. False	91. True	98. False
78. True	85. True	92. False	99. True
79. False	86. False	93. False	100. True

Match the Followings

Part A

1.	F	6.	C
2.	A	7.	B
3.	D	8.	I
4.	E	9.	J
5.	G	10.	H

Part B

1.	D	6.	G
2.	E	7.	H
3.	F	8.	B
4.	C	9.	J
5.	A	10.	I

Part C

1.	B	6.	G
2.	C	7.	I
3.	D	8.	F
4.	A	9.	E
5.	J	10.	H

Part D

1.	J	6.	E
2.	I	7.	D
3.	H	8.	G
4.	F	9.	A
5.	C	10.	B

Part E

1.	H	6.	C
2.	A	7.	D
3.	F	8.	G
4.	E	9.	J
5.	B	10.	I

Part F

1.	H	6.	E
2.	G	7.	C
3.	I	8.	J
4.	F	9.	B
5.	D	10.	A

Part G

1.	D	6.	I
2.	E	7.	J
3.	F	8.	C
4.	G	9.	B
5.	H	10.	A

Chapter 4

Environmental Hygiene

MULTIPLE CHOICE QUESTIONS

1. **The sum total of all external conditions and influences effecting life and development of living being is known as:**

   (a) Environment (b) Ecosystem

   (c) Atmosphere (d) Biome

2. **All the following are regarded as physical environmental hazard except:**

   (a) Température (b) Humidity

   (c) Radiation (d) Stress

3. **The amount of body water in human varies with:**

   (a) Age (b) Adiposity

   (c) Sex (d) All of above

4. **The palatability of water is generally considered to be good with TDS level of:**

   (a) 600mg/L (b) 1000mg/L

   (c) 1200mg/L (d) 100mg/L

5. **The permissible limit of lead in drinking water as per WHO guideline should be:**
   (a) 0.01mg/L (b) 0.05mg/L
   (c) 1.0mg/L (d) 10.0mg/L

6. **The most common way of absorption of lead is:**
   (a) Inhalation (b) Skin absorption
   (c) Ingestion (d) All of above

7. **The minimum recommended standard for mercury in drinking water by WHO is:**
   (a) 0.01mg/L (b) 0.001mg/
   (c) 0.5mg/LL (d) 100mg/L

8. **The minimum permissible limit for arsenic in drinking water by WHO is:**
   (a) 0.01mg/L (b) 0.05mg/L
   (c) 0.001mg/L (d) 100mg/L

9. **Which one of following in higher concentration is intestinal irritant:**
   (a) Iron (b) Copper
   (c) Arsenic (d) Lead

10. **The presence of garlic odour in expired breath, falling of hair, rough and dry skin and reddening of eye indicates:**
    (a) Zinc toxicity (b) Copper toxicity
    (c) Arsenic toxicity (d) Lead toxicity

11. **Staining of laundry and sanitary ware occurs if concentration of_______ is beyond permissible limit.**
    (a) Copper (b) Iron
    (c) Manganèse (d) All of above

12. **Arsenic comes in water from agricultural practices. Which one of following is a source of arsenic:**
    (a) Weedicide (b) Fungicide
    (c) Sheep dip (d) All of above

13. Lead is toxic for______ nervous system:

(a) Peripheral (b) Central

(c) Both (a) and (b) (d) None of above

14. Dieldrin is used as ______ in agricultural practices.

(a) Weedicide (b) Fungicide

(c) Insecticide (d) Herbicide

15. Dieldrin remains suspended in the air for long time and can reach the body of animal and man through

(a) Food (b) Water

(c) Inhalation (d) All of above

16. All the following end products are produced by aerobic decomposition of organic matter except:

(a) Water (b) Carbon dioxide

(c) Methane (d) Amonia

17. All the following diseases are transmitted by inhalation of droplet nuclei except:

(a) Typhoid (b) Tuberculosis

(c) Q fever (d) Influenza

18. Which of the following water borne disease has been eradicated from the country?

(a) Cholera (b) Leptospirosis

(c) Guinea worm disease (d) Schistosomiasis

19. Which one of the following is most important component of greenhouse effect:

(a) CO_2 (b) H_2O

(c) NO_2 (d) CH_3

20. All the following water borne diseases are transmitted by penetration of skin except:

(a) Leptospirosis (b) Schistosomiasis

(c) Cholera (d) Guinea worm disease

21. Which component is essential for dental health :

(a) Chloride (b) Nitrate

(c) Lead (d) Flouride

22. Which of the following gas imparts rotten egg odour to water:

(a) SO_2 (b) H_2S

(c) NO_2 (d) CH_3

23. The determination of _______ is one of the best methods for assessing biologically oxidisable organic matter.

(a) DO (b) BOD

(c) COD (d) None of above

24. The methods used for removal of temporary hardness of water is/are

(a) Boiling (b) Addition of lime

(c) Both (a) and (b) (d) None of above

25. Dechlorination of treated water is done by adding

(a) SO_2 (b) Sodiumthiosulphate

(c) Both (a) and (b) (d) None of above

26. The presence of free residual chlorine is essential for atleast _______hour.

(a) 15 minutes (b) One

(c) half (d) Two

27. The water which comes above the first impervious layer is called as

(a) Surface water (b) Shallow well water

(c) Ground water (d) Rain water

28. Which type of water supply system is most reliable and economic?

(a) Gravity system (b) Pumping system

(c) Combined (d) None

29. The disease which is transmitted by penetration of intact skin while working in water is:

(a) Leptospirosis (b) Schistosomiasis

(c) Meliodosis (d) Fascioliasis

30. All the following organisms belong to coliform group except:

(a) *Proteus* (b) *E. coli*

(c) *Enterobacter* (d) *Citrobacter*

31. Which one of the following is non-faecal Atypical) coliform?

(a) *E. coli* type IV (b) E. coli type II

(c) Both (a) and (b) (d) None of above

32. All the following are examples of surface water except:

(a) River (b) Spring

(c) Seawater (d) Streams

33. The highest desirable level of hardness in drinking water as per WHO should be:

(a) 50ppm (b) 100ppm

(c) 150ppm (d) 200ppm

34. Permutit process is performed with sodium permutit which is a complex compound containing following except:

(a) Sodium (b) Silver

(c) Aluminium (d) Silica

35. All the followings are examples of filters that are used for purification of water on small scale except:

(a) Pasteur chamberland filter (b) Seitz filter

(c) Berkfeld filter (d) Katadyn filter

36. The filter candles of berkfeld filter are made up of:

(a) Porcelain (b) Kaolin

(c) Nitrocellulose (d) Silver ion

37. The______ quality of filtered water is very high in case of slow sand filter:

(a) Physical (b) Chemical

(c) Bacteriological (d) All of above

38. The vital layer is said to be the heart of slow sand filter because it:

(a) Removes the organic matter

(b) Oxidizes ammoniacal nitrogen

(c) Retains bacteria (d) All of above

39. When 'loss of head' exceeds _______, it is uneconomical to run slow sand filter.

(a) 1.0 meter (b) 1.3 meter

(c) 1.5 meter (d) 2.0 meter

40. The dose of alum for chemical coagulation of raw water in rapid sand filtration depends upon:

(a) Turbidity (b) Colour

(c) pH value (d) All of above

41. The treatment stage(s) that precedes filtration process in rapid sand filter is/are

(a) Coagulation (b) Flocculation

(c) Sedimentation (d) All of above

42. The reagent used for determining efficiency of chlorination

(a) Chlortex (b) Orthotoludine

(c) Eriochrome black T (d) Both (a) and (b)

43. The test which can detect both free and combined chlorine in water

(a) Methylene blue reduction test (b) Chlortex test

(c) Orthotolidine test (d) Resazurin test

44. The most widely used disinfection method of swimming pool is:

(a) Chlorination (b) UV irradiation

(c) SO_2 treatment (d) Ozonization

45. Which one of the following is most strong virucidal agent?

(a) Chlorine
(b) Iodine
(c) UV rays
(d) Ozone

46. The organism that converts ammonia to nitrate in water is:

(a) Crenothrix
(b) Gallionella
(c) Nitrosomonas
(d) Nitrobacter

47. The role of iron bacteria in water is to:

(a) Synthesize iron
(b) Decompose iron
(c) Metabolize iron
(d) Abstract iron

48. The factor that has marked effect on BOD estimation of water is:

(a) Acid and Alkali
(b) Free chlorine
(c) Salinity
(d) Toxic metals

49. The 5 days BOD value is only a portion of total BOD and it amounts to about:

(a) 50 per cent
(b) 70 per cent -80 per cent
(c) 60 per cent
(d) 80 per cent -90 per cent

50. The BOD value of treated water should be:

(a) 30 mg/L
(b) 50 mg/L
(c) 100 mg/L
(d) 250 mg/L

51. The COD value of treated water should be:

(a) 30 mg/L
(b) 50 mg/L
(c) 100 mg/L
(d) 250 mg/L

52. The activated sludge should be mixed in effluent of primary sedimentation tank for biological treatment in portion of:

(a) 5-10 per cent
(b) 20-30 per cent
(c) 40 per cent
(d) 50 per cent

53. Wastewater can be used for following purpose:

(a) Public water supply
(b) Rehabilitation of natural ecosystem
(c) Both (a) and (b)
(d) None of above

54. The grit chamber is a long chamber having the dimension of:

(a) 10-20 m (b) 40m

(c) 30 m (d) 50 m

55. The sewage passes through grit chamber with a constant velocity of about:

(a) 10 cm/sec (b) 20 cm/sec

(c) 30 cm/sec (d) 40 cm/sec

56. The sewage is detained in grit chamber for a period of:

(a) 10-20 sec (b) 30- 60 sec

(c) 2-3 hours (d) 6-8 hours

57. The detention period of sewage in primary sedimentation tank is:

(a) 2-3 hours (b) 4-5 hours

(c) 6-8 hours (d) 2-3 week

58. The sewage is detained in aeration tank for a period of:

(a) 2-3 hours (b) 4-5 hours

(c) 6-8 hours (d) 2-3 week

59. The detention period of sewage in secondary sedimentation tank is:

(a) 2-3 hours (b) 4-5 hours

(c) 6-8 hours (d) 2-3 week

60. The velocity of sewage passing through primary sedimentation tank is about:

(a) 10-20cm/min (b) 20-30cm/min

(c) 30-60 cm/min (d) 30-60 cm/sec

61. The end products of aerobic decomposition of sewage are:

(a) CO_2 and H_2O (b) NH_3 and SO_4

(c) Nitrate and nitrite (d) All of above

62. The end product of anaerobic decomposition of sewage is/are:

(a) CO_2 and H_2 (b) NH_3

(c) Methane (d) All of above

63. The word 'Grey Water' is synonymously used for:

(a) Sewage (b) Sullage

(c) Sludge (d) Slurry

64. The atmospheric zone found immediately above the earth is:

(a) Troposphere (b) Mesosphere

(c) Stratosphere (d) Thermosphere

65. Which of the following gas is not present in thermosphere?

(a) Ozone (b) Oxygen

(c) Nascent oxygen (d) Nitrogen oxide

66. The general level of air pollution is indicated by the presence of _______ in the air.

(a) Smoke (b) SPM

(c) SO_2 (d) All of above

67. Which source is responsible for largest emission of Cadmium in atmosphere?

(a) Steel industry (b) Volcanic eruption

(c) Waste incineration (d) All of above

68. Which of the following is consumed through tobacco?

(a) Cadmium (b) SO_2

(c) Lead (d) CO

69. Carbon monoxide is a _______ type of air pollutant.

(a) Irritant (b) Nonirritant

(c) Particulate (d) None of above

70. The most common air borne chemical contaminant is:

(a) Lead (b) Silica

(c) Asbestos (d) Mercury

71. Burning of fossil fuels and wood releases the pollutant like:

(a) CO (b) Hydrocarbon

(c) SO_2 (d) All of above

72. Acid rain is caused by following gases:

(a) CO_2, SO_2, NO_2 (b) SO_2,CO_2,O_3

(c) SO_2,CO_2 (d) CO, SO_2, NO_2

73. Which one of the following is known as bagasse?

(a) Coal dust (b) Sugarcane dust

(c) Cotton dust (d) Asbestos dust

74. The hazardous effect of dust depend on which factor:

(a) Size (b) Concentration

(c) Duration of exposure (d) All of above

75. Chernobyl disaster was the outcome of :

(a) Leakage of toxic gas (b) Leakage of radioactivity

(c) Formation of smog (d) Coal dust explosion

76. The potency of radiation is measured in:

(a) Roentgen (b) Rem

(c) Rad (d) All of above

77. Example of anthropogenic source of air pollution is:

(a) Volcanic eruption (b) Dust storm

(c) Nuclear explosion (d) Forest fire

78. The radioactive element present in man's terrestrial environment, is/are:

(a) Radium (b) Thorium

(c) Uranium (d) All of above

79. The electromagnetic radiation which is non-ionizing:

(a) UV rays (b) Gamma rays

(c) Infrared rays (d) Both (a) and (c)

80. The greatest man made source of radiation exposure to general population is:

(a) UV rays (b) Gamma rays

(c) X-rays (d) None of above

81. Which of the following non-ionizing radiation has highest wavelength?

(a) UV rays (b) Infrared rays

(c) Visible sunlight (d) Microwave radiation

82. All the following are examples of corpuscular radiations except one:

(a) Gamma rays (b) Beta particles

(c) Alpha particle (d) Protons

83. The activities concerning animal welfare in India are regulated through provisions of:

(a) Cattle Trespass Act

(b) Prevention of cruelty to animals Act

(c) Goshala Act

(d) Animal welfare Act

84. The Prevention of Cruelty to Animals Act provides protection to the animals from:

(a) Cruelty (b) Disease

(c) Infirmity (d) All of above

85. National Environmental Engineering Research Institute is situated at:

(a) Kanpur (b) Delhi

(c) Mumbai (d) Nagpur

86. The first UN conference on human environment was held in:

(a) Stockholm (b) Geneva

(c) Atlanta (d) Rio De Generio

87. During quarantine period, animals are subjected to:

(a) Screening for disease (b) De-worming

(b) Immunization (d) All of above

88. Quaternary Amonium Compound (QAC) can be used to disinfect:

(a) Animal houses (b) Animal discharge

(c) Dairy utensils (d) All of above

89. Which of the following is highly effective against bacterial spores?

(a) Bleaching powder (b) Cresol

(c) Lysol (d) QAC

90. Which one is more practical to check the aerial infection in animal houses?

(a) UV irradiation (b) Fumigation

(c) Flaming (d) Ozonization

91. The concentration of caustic soda at which it is highly effective disinfectant for animal houses following the outbreak of FMD, swine fever or other contagious disease is:

(a) 2 per cent (b) 3 per cent

(c) 5 per cent (d) 10 per cent

92. The noise level that can damage tympanic membrane is:

(a) 160 dB (b) 200dB

(c) 100 dB (d) All of above

93. The non-auditory effects of noise pollution is/are:

(a) Interference in speech (b) Mental Efficiency loss

(c) Annoyance (d) All of above

94. Segregation of new animals before their addition to original healthy stock is called as:

(a) Quarantine (b) Isolation

(c) Elimination (d) Eradication

95. The quarantine period usually corresponds to______ period of disease:

(a) Incubation (b) Duration

(c) Convalescent (d) All of above

96. Internationally accepted diseases specified by WHO that require quarantine:

(a) Plague
(b) Small pox
(c) Cholera
(d) All of above

97. Internationally accepted vector-borne diseases specified by WHO for quarantine is/are:

(a) Yellow fever
(b) Typhus fever
(c) Relapsing fever
(d) All of above

98. Cyanide may be found in drinking water primarily as a consequence of_______ contamination:

(a) Agricultural
(b) Industrial
(c) Urban waste
(d) All of above

99. Silicosis is encountered in the workers employed in:

(a) Mine
(b) Pottery and ceramic industry
(c) Construction work
(d) All of above

100. Sir Joseph Lister, a pioneer in antiseptic surgery, introduced _______ to sterilize surgical equipment and to clean the wound:

(a) Carbolic acid
(b) Benzoic acid
(c) Acriflavin
(d) Alcohol

FILL IN THE BLANKS

1. The science of health that contributes to healthful living is called as_______.
2. The sum total of all the conditions and influences affecting the life and development of any living being is termed as _______.
3. 'World Environment day' is celebrated on _______ June.
4. Animal and plant life of a specific area is termed as _______.

5. The body of healthy animal contains water and proteins in a ratio of _______.
6. The water of _______and _______ (water sources) is considered wholesome and safe for drinking.
7. The process of making a well leak proof is called as _______.
8. The pH of drinking water should be _______ according to WHO guidelines.
9. Flat and insipid taste of water may be attributed to extremely low concentration of _______.
10. Ground water reaching the earth surface on account of its own hydrostatic pressure is called _______.
11. When pH of water is _______, it interferes with efficiency of chlorination.
12. Turbidity in water is caused by _______ and _______ types of impurities.
13. Distillation is used as a method of choice for water purification in _______.
14. _______ is the internationally accepted bacterial indicator for detecting recent sewage pollution of water.
15. Presence of _______ (bacteria) in water indicates that pollution is long standing.
16. Coliforms that are able to grow at _______ (temperature), are called fecal coliform.
17. Name the table used to estimate the Most Probable Number (MPN) of coliforms _______.
18. As per BIS, number of coliform in drinking water should be _______.
19. According to WHO's guidelines, number of coliforms in drinking water should be _______.
20. Confirmatory coliform test is also known as_______.
21. The chlorine left in water after satisfying chlorine demand is called as _______.

22. Chlorine may be applied either in _______or _______ form.
23. The point at which chlorine demand of water is met is called _______ chlorination.
24. After chlorination, _______ of residual chlorine should be left in water.
25. The contact period for chlorination should be_______.
26. Blue color of water after addition of chlortex reagent indicates that _______ chlorine is present in water.
27. The disinfecting action of chlorine in water is mainly due to_______.
28. The most commonly used chemical agent for chlorination of water is _______.
29. When acidic water passes from lead pipes, it dissolves some amount of lead. This action of acidic water is called as_______.
30. The disadvantage of chlorine treatment is the formation of _______, if water is having high organic matter.
31. Dechlorination of water on large scale can be done by addition of _______.
32. The reagent used for estimation of residual chlorine in water is _______.
33. The formation of _______ oxidizes the organic matter and kills the microorganism on ozonization.
34. Algal growth in pond water can be removed by _______.
35. The hardness of water caused by carbonate and bicarbonate salt, is called as _______.
36. Name the dye used in hardness indicator tablet is _______.
37. The permanent hardness in water is due to_______ and _______ of calcium and magnesium.
38. Removal of temporary hardness could be achieved by adding _______ in water.
39. Permanent hardness can be removed by _______ method.

40. The deposition of calcium and magnesium carbonate in kettle or boiler is known as _______.
41. The quantity of oxygen required by bacteria for biochemical degradation of organic matter under aerobic condition is referred as _______.
42. The amount of oxygen required for chemical oxidation of organic matter is referred as _______.
43. BOD determination is the measurement of dissolved oxygen before and after _______ of incubation at _______.
44. The chemical oxidation demand of the organic matter can be measured by using a strong chemical oxidant such as _______.
45. The un-reacted potassium dichromate is back titrated with _______ for COD estimation.
46. Presence of a foreign substances in water/air/environment in an amount injurious to health is called _______.
47. The practice of disinfectant sprays on wound was first introduced by _______.
48. Germicidal power of disinfectant can be estimated by determining _______.
49. The process of removal of colloidal impurities from water is called _______ while the process used for removal of coarse suspended impurities is called_______.
50. Give two examples of coagulating agents for water _______, _______.
51. The depth of sand layer in case of slow sand filter should be around _______ inches, however in case of rapid sand filter, it should be _______ inches.
52. There are two types of rapid sand filter; one is _______ type and other is_______ type.
53. The rate of filtration in rapid sand filter is _______ m^3/m^2/hour.
54. Backwashing of rapid sand filter is achieved by reversing the flow of _______ and adding _______.
55. Rapid sand filter removes all the particles and impurities that have been trapped in_______ through flocculation.

56. As the water flows through filter medium, the floc material is retained by ______.
57. The device which measures the bed resistance or loss of head in slow sand filter is called ______.
58. Water should be free from ______ for efficient disinfection by UV irradiation.
59. The filter candle is made up of ______ in Chamberland filter.
60. The bacteria coming in contact with the surface of Katadyn filter are killed by ______ action of silver ion.
61. The problem of fluorosis is common in ______ and ______ grazing on land near aluminium, fertilizer plant and brick klins.
62. Two water borne diseases, which are transmitted by skin penetration are ______ and ______.
63. The most important gas responsible for ozone layer depletion is______.
64. Pneumococcosis caused by inhalation of moldy hay or grain dust is called as ______. It is caused by the growth of actinomycetes known as ______.
65. The size of expiratory droplets is about ______, however the size of droplet nuclei ranges between ______.
66. The air pollutants are classified into ______ and ______ on the basis of physicochemical characteristics.
67. The presence of large number of microbes like bacteria, viruses, fungi and protozoa in the atmosphere is called as ______.
68. Small gas borne particle mainly composed of carbon in air is called ______.
69. The agglomeration of fine carbon particles containing hydrocarbons and mineral matter is called ______.
70. Smoke mixed with dust is called as ______.
71. Release of substances into the atmosphere from natural and man-made sources is called ______.

72. The technique of collecting the air sample through a slit on the surface of liquid media is called______.
73. The device used to collect the air particle on media is named as _______.
74. The device used to collect the air sample on the basis of particle size of the pollutant is called _______.
75. The smoke content of the air is expressed as _______ unit per 1000 linear feet of air sample.
76. The atmospheric zone which is characterized by very high temperature is called _______.
77. Rad means_______.
78. The radiation energy received per unit of material exposed is measured in_______.
79. The effect of radiation on biological material is measured in _______.
80. The radiation unit rad is now replaced by _______.
81. The radiation unit rem is now replaced by _______.
82. The release of radioactivity into the atmosphere from nuclear explosion is called _______.
83. Ionizing radiation may be broadly divided into two main groups; _______ and _______.
84. The biological effects of ionizing radiation may be divided into two; _______ and _______.
85. The radioactive gases released in atmosphere are _______ and_______.
86. An enclosure maintained by public authority for confining stray or homeless animal is called _______.
87. The animals that roam about freely and create nuisance for the community are called _______ animals.
88. The animals which are dead or lying on the ground are called_______ animals.
89. The activity of stray animals in India is regulated by the _______ act, 1921.

90. The agency that has a mandate of animal welfare activities in India is _______.
91. Waste- matter containing solid and liquid excreta derived from farmyard washings, houses roads and factories is called_______.
92. _______ is the wastewater from houses unmixed with human excreta.
93. The amount of manure produced per day per cattle unit in a normal course is about _______.
94. The sewage contains about _______ water with organic and inorganic matter.
95. One million tons of sewage produces _______ of sludge.
96. The organic matter that settles down in the bottom of primary sedimentation tank of sewage treatment plant is called _______.
97. The organic matter that settles down in the bottom of final sedimentation tank is called _______.
98. Anaerobic breakdown of animal waste is a biochemical process which is commonly known as _______.
99. The major gases released from the process of methanogenesis are _______ and _______.
100. The biological effects of noise pollution are classified into two; _______ and _______ effect.

MARK TRUE/FALSE

1. Soft water is neither good for drinking nor for washing.
2. The mammalian body contains 70-75 per cent water while, new-born baby has about 90 per cent of water.
3. Artificial ultraviolet irradiation is an important physical method which is routinely used to purify large quantity of water.
4. The presence of ammonia in water is a strong indicator of its recent pollution with sewage.

5. Iron is a frequent constituent of potable water but in large quantity, it imparts bitter taste to the water.
6. Wholesome water should not contain more than1 mg/L of fluoride.
7. The presence of copper in water increases the corrosion of galvanized iron and steel fitting.
8. Water containing Manganese beyond permissible limit may appear opalescent and develop greasy film on boiling.
9. The pH of water should be neutral for making chlorination process efficient.
10. High test hypochlorite is more stable than bleaching powder and deteriorates much less on storage.
11. Non-fecal coliforms are thermotolerant.
12. Fecal coliform count in untreated water should not be more than 10/100ml as per BIS.
13. The number of coliform in water is about one tenth that of faecal *Streptococci.*
14. *E. coli* (Type1) are the true (typical) faecal coliforms because they have ability to produce indole at 44°C, however atypical *E. coli* do not produce indole from tryptophan at 44°C.
15. Atypical *E. coli* do not ferment lactose to produce acid and gas at 44°C.
16. The presence of *Streptococcus faecalis* in water indicates that pollution is long standing.
17. Coliform do not multiply in water but survive longer than other enteropathogens.
18. The iron bacteria of water cannot be destroyed by chlorination.
19. Polio and infectious hepatitis virus can be easily destroyed by chlorination.
20. Chemical oxygen demand estimates both degradable and non-degradable organic matter.

21. BOD is the best measure for checking the level of organic pollution and assessing purification capacity of streams.
22. About 90 per cent of suspended impurities in water settle down in 24 hour during storage by gravity.
23. Scrapping of sand bed is needed more frequently in rapid sand filter than in slow sand filter.
24. The rapid sand filters require larger area than slow sand filter.
25. The water drawn from the reservoir should first be treated with chemical coagulant in case of slow sand filter.
26. Venturimeter is an important component of rapid sand filter.
27. When the loss of head in slow sand filter exceeds 1.3 meter, it is uneconomical to run the filter.
28. The cost of construction of rapid sand filter is cheaper than that of slow sand filter.
29. The depth of sand layer should be more in case of rapid sand filter than in slow sand filter.
30. The layer of graded gravel below the sand bed is needed to provide support to the sand bed and permit the filtered water to move freely.
31. The height of water column should be more in rapid sand filter to maintain the pressure above the filter bed.
32. Back washing is needed for cleaning of slow sand filter.
33. Slow sand filter is said to be ripened when filter's sand bed is coated with organisms.
34. Ripening of slow sand filter occurs after a period of 12 hours.
35. Rapid sand filter has little effect on taste and smell and dissolved impurities of water unless activated carbon is included in the medium.
36. The sum of chlorine demand plus free residual chlorine constitutes the correct dose of chlorine to be applied.
37. Chlorination is used as a supplement, not as a substitute to sand filtration.

38. Chloramine require long contact period because it is a slow bactericidal agent.
39. Chloramine is affected to a greater extent by presence of organic matter.
40. Although action of chloramines is slower than chlorine but it gives more persistent type of residual chlorine.
41. Orthotolidine reacts more rapidly with combined chlorine than free chlorine.
42. Very soft water is good from dietic point of view.
43. Very hard water is not considered good for domestic purposes like drinking and washing.
44. Ozonization is usually employed in combination with chlorination.
45. The ozone dose required for treatment of drinking water varies from 0.2 to 1.5 mg/L.
46. One mili equivalents/L of hardness is equal to 150 ppm of $CaCO_3$.
47. Sodium carbonate can remove both temporary and permanent hardness from water.
48. The maximum permissible limit of hardness for consumer is 300- 600 mg/L.
49. In large scale treatment of water supplies, the permutit process is used for removal of hardness.
50. Smoke or air test is done for leakage of pipelines.
51. Mercury mainly damages the nervous system and kidneys.
52. Inorganic mercury mainly targets central nervous system whereas organic mercury targets kidney.
53. Expired air has reduced oxygen concentration and increased carbon dioxide concentration.
54. Ozone shield is found in troposphere.
55. Ozone shield mainly protects the earth surface from infrared radiation.
56. Green house effect is a desirable phenomenon.

57. Effect of radiation on biological material is measured in rad.
58. The radiation unit Roentgen is now replaced by Coulomb/kg (C/kg).
59. The term ionizing radiation is applied to radiation which has ability to penetrate tissues and deposit its energy within them.
60. The wavelength of non-ionizing radiations is shorter than ionizing radiations.
61. The half life of Cesium is 28 yrs, while half life of Strontium is 30 years.
62. Alpha particles are 10 times as harmful as X rays.
63. Radon gas is released in the atmosphere by radioactive decay occurring in earth crust.
64. Largest natural source of methane emission on earth is wetland.
65. Indicators of air pollution are fog, mist, smog, smoke *etc.*
66. Aerosol refers to dispersion of solid and liquid particle into gaseous media like smoke or fog to form a colloidal form.
67. Mist refers to moderate dispersion of minute droplets in the atmosphere.
68. Fog denotes aerosols in which dispersed phase is water.
69. Particulate pollutants are solid and liquid particles, suspended in the atmosphere, which are larger than single molecule but smaller than 500 micron.
70. Burning of fossil fuel and wood releases the pollutant like CO, SO_2, Oxides of nitrogen and hydrocarbon.
71. The droplet nuclei are primary mode of spread of a variety of contagious diseases.
72. About 99 per cent gaseous mass is found in mesosphere of the atmosphere.
73. Silicosis is commonly seen in workers employed in metal grinding.
74. Bagassosis is caused by inhalation of cotton dust.

75. Silicosis is caused by inhalation of dust containing free silica or silicon dioxide.
76. Carbon monoxide is a good example of non-irritant pollutant.
77. In animal houses, main irritating gases are methane and ammonia.
78. The maximum permissible limit of noise for human being is 85db.
79. The thermocomfort zone is the temperature range within which animal are capable of giving maximum performance.
80. An adult sheep can withstand in température range of -7 to 30° C.
81. The thermocomfort zone for adult pig ranges between 4- 30°C.
82. The comfort zone for European cattle is about 0- 20°C.
83. The thermocomfort zone for broilers is 18-21°C.
84. The term climate denotes short term atmospheric condition of a region.
85. The critical température leading to decline in milk yield of tropical cattle is more than 38°C.
86. An average daily requirement of water for dairy cattle should be 110 litre per head.
87. An average daily requirement of water for a horse under average stable feeding is 72 liter per head.
88. Sewage is said to be strong if the amount of suspended solids excède 500mg/litre.
89. Activated sludge is rich in anaerobic bacteria.
90. Screening chamber removes heavier solid matter from the sewage.
91. The grit chamber is used to remove all the organic impurities after primary sedimentation.
92. Activated sludge treatment involves anaerobic breakdown of organic matter.
93. Slurry from a dairy herd of 50 cows and 50 sows can cause pollution load that is equivalent to that of a village of 1000 people.
94. The term dry weather flow is used to denote average amount of air flowing through ventilation system in animal house.

95. The noise level between 60-70 decibel represents calm environment.
96. Non-enveloped viruses are unstable in dry conditions but survive better at relative high humidity.
97. High relative humidity allows survival of the viruses with lipoprotein envelope.
98. The activities of goshalas are regulated by cattle trespass Act.
99. National Eco Development Board was established in 1981 with an aim to develop wasteland.
100. The activities regarding environmental pollution control in India are coordinated by NEERI.

MATCHING TYPE QUESTIONS

Part A

Column – A		*Column – B*
1. Copper sulphate	(__)	a. Smog disaster
2. Aluminium sulphate	(__)	b. Methyl isocyanide gas tragedy
3. Bleaching powder	(__)	c. Coliform
4. *Gallionella*	(__)	d. Iron bacteria
5. *Klebsiella*	(__)	e. Trihalomethane
6. Bhopal	(__)	f. Radiation disaster
7. Chernobyl	(__)	g. cleaning of mud, silt or color
8. London	(__)	h. Reduces algal growth
9. Bioshere	(__)	i. Crust of earth
10. Lithosphere	(__)	j. Region of earth containing soil, air, water

Part B

Column – A		Column – B
1. Schmutz decke	(__)	a. Aquaguard
2. Farmer's lung	(__)	b. Catadyn bead type sterilizer
3. Black lung	(__)	c. Coal dust
4. Trickle filter	(__)	d. Sewage treatment
5. Meta filter	(__)	e. Coagulation
6. Ultra-care water filter	(__)	f. Biological film
7. Colloidal impurities	(__)	g. Hay dust
8. Suspended impurities	(__)	h. Sedimentation
9. Coliform	(__)	i. Recent sewage pollution
10. *Cl. perfringes*	(__)	j. Long standing sewage pollution

Part C

Column – A		Column – B
1. Plankton	(__)	a. Toxic Chemical
2. Physical pollutant	(__)	b. Rapid sand filter
3. Industrial pollutant	(__)	c. Radioactive substance
4. Mechanical Filter	(__)	d. Benthal organism
5. Biological Filter	(__)	e. Slow sand filter
6. Turbidity	(__)	f. Potassium dichromate
7. Chlorine dose	(__)	g. Naphalometer
8. COD	(__)	h. Horrock's apparatus
9. Water color	(__)	i. Nessler's reagent
10. Ammonia in water	(__)	j. Platinum-cobalt scale

Part D

Column – A		*Column – B*
1. Anthracosis	(__)	a. Iron dust
2. Siderosis	(__)	b. Sugarcane dust
3. Bagassosis	(__)	c. Cotton fibre dust
4. Byssinosis	(__)	d. Iron
5. Plumbism	(__)	e. Coal dust
6. Chalaybeat	(__)	f. Dental carries
7. Droplet nuclei	(__)	g. Diphtheria
8. Droplet infection	(__)	h. Less than 10µ
9. Knackeries	(__)	i. Biological film
10. Vital layer	(__)	j. Veterinaryian certificate

Part D

Column – A		*Column – B*
1. Hard water	(__)	a. Lead poisoning
2. Ferrobacteria	(__)	b. Depleted by Freon
3. Ozone	(__)	c. Weil's disease
4. Flurosis	(__)	d. Jaundice
5. Acidic water	(__)	e. Dysentry
6. Leptospirosis	(__)	f. Swimmer's itch
7. Infectious hepatitis	(__)	g. Rice water stool
8. Vibrio cholerae	(__)	h. Calculi formation
9. *Entamoeba histolytica*	(__)	i. Dental dystrophy
10. Systosomiasis	(__)	j. *Crenothrix* spp.

Part E

Column – A		*Column – B*
1. *Gallionella*	(__)	a. Slimy layer
2. *Crenothrix*	(__)	b. Incrustation
3. Ozonization	(__)	c. Ponds
4. Copper sulfate	(__)	d. Swimming pool
5. Orthotolidine	(__)	e. Chlorine dose
6. Horrock's apparatus	(__)	f. Residual chlorine
7. *E. coli* type I	(__)	g. Non-fecal coliform
8. *E. coli* type II	(__)	h. True coliform
9. Patterson's filter	(__)	i. Pressure type rapid sand filer
10. Candy's filter	(__)	j. Gravity type rapid sand filer.

Part F

Column – A		*Column – B*
1. Incipid taste of water	(__)	a. Calcium hypochloride
2. Bitter taste of water	(__)	b. Calcium hydroxide
3. Musty odour	(__)	c. Calcium oxide
4. Rotten egg odour	(__)	d. Color of water
5. SPM	(__)	e. Turbidity of water
6. Bleaching powder	(__)	f. Boiling
7. Slaked lime	(__)	g. Chlorination
8. Quick lime	(__)	h. Fungal growth (Decaying vegetable matter)
9. TCU	(__)	i. H_2S (Decomposing sewage)
10. NTU	(__)	j. Measure of air pollution

ANSWERS

Multiple Choice Questions

1.(a)	2.(d)	3.(d)	4.(a)	5.(b)	6.(a)	7.(b)
8.(b)	9.(c)	10.(c)	11.(d)	12.(d)	13.(c)	14.(c)
15.(d)	16.(c)	17.(a)	18.(c)	19.(a)	20.(c)	21.(d)
22.(b)	23.(b)	24.(c)	25.(c)	26.(b)	27.(b)	28.(a)
29.(a)	30.(a)	31.(c)	32.(b)	33.(b)	34.(b)	35.(b)
36.(b)	37.(d)	38.(d)	39.(b)	40.(d)	41.(d)	42.(d)
43.(c)	44.(a)	45.(d)	46.(c)	47.(d)	48.(a)	49.(b)
50.(a)	51.(d)	52.(b)	53.(c)	54.(a)	55.(c)	56.(b)
57.(c)	58.(c)	59.(a)	60.(c)	61.(d)	62.(d)	63.(b)
64.(a)	65.(a)	66.(d)	67.(d)	68.(a)	69.(b)	70.(a)
71.(d)	72.(a)	73.(b)	74.(d)	75.(b)	76.(d)	77.(c)
78.(d)	79.(d)	80.(c)	81.(a)	82.(a)	83.(b)	84.(d)
85.(d)	86.(a)	87.(d)	88.(a)	89.(a)	90.(b)	91.(a)
92.(a)	93.(d)	94.(a)	95.(d)	96.(d)	97.(d)	98.(b)
99.(d)	100.(a)					

Fill in the Blanks

1. Hygiene
2. Environment
3. 5th June
4. Biota
5. 4:1
6. Deep well and spring
7. Steining
8. 6.5-8.5
9. TDS
10. Spring
11. Alkaline (8)
12. Colloidal and suspended
13. Ship, Laboratory, Arabian country
14. *E. coli*
15. *Clostridium perfringens*
16. 44°C
17. Macrady's table
18. Less than 10/100ml
19. Zero/100 ml

20. Eijkman test
21. Residual chlorine
22. Gaseous or suspension
23. Breakpoint
24. 0.1- 0.2mg/ml
25. 30 min.
26. 1.0 ppm
27. Hypochlorous acid
28. Bleaching powder
29. Plumbosolvency
30. Trihelomethane
31. SO_2
32. Chlortex
33. Nascent oxygen
34. Copper sulfate
35. Temporary hardness
36. Eriochrome black T
37. chloride and sulphates
38. Lime
39. Ion exchange
40. Furring
41. BOD
42. COD
43. 5 days, 20°C
44. Potassium dichromate
45. Ferrous ammonium sulphate
46. Pollution
47. Joseph Lister
48. Inhibition coefficient
49. Coagulation, screening
50. Alum, Ferrous Sulphate
51. 36-60, 30-36
52. Gravity, pressure
53. 5-15
54. Water, Compressed air
55. Floc
56. Sand matrix
57. Venturimeter
58. Turbidity
59. Porcelain
60. Oligodynamic
61. Cattle and sheep
62. Weil's disease, Swimmer's itch
63. CFC
64. Farmer's lung, *Micropolyspora faeni*
65. 10 μ, 1-10 μ
66. Particulate and gaseous
67. Germ cloud
68. Smoke
69. Soot
70. Smust
71. Emission
72. Impingement
73. Slit sampler
74. Sieve sampler
75. Coh
76. Thermosphere
77. Radiation absorbed dose
78. Rad

79. Rem
80. Grey (Gy)
81. Sivert (Sy)
82. Fall out
83. Electromagnetic and Corpuscular radiation
84. Somatic and genetic effects
85. Radon, thoron
86. Pound
87. Stray
88. Fallen
89. cattle trespass
90. Animal welfare board
91. Sewage
92. Sullage
93. 40 kg
94. 99 per cent
95. 15-20 tons
96. Sludge
97. Activated sludge
98. Methanogenesis
99. Methane, CO_2
100. Auditory and non-auditory

MARK TRUE/FALSE

1. False
2. True
3. False
4. True
5. True
6. True
7. True
8. False
9. True
10. True
11. False
12. False
13. False
14. True
15. False
16. False
17. True
18. False
19. False
20. True
21. True
22. True
23. False
24. False
25. False
26. False
27. True
28. False
29. False
30. True
31. True
32. False
33. True
34. True
35. True
36. True
37. True
38. True
39. False
40. True
41. False
42. False
43. True
44. True
45. True
46. False
47. True
48. True
49. True
50. True
51. True
52. False
53. True
54. False
55. False
56. True
57. False
58. True
59. True
60. False
61. True
62. True
63. True
64. True
65. True
66. True
67. True
68. True

69. True	77. True	85. True	93. True
70. True	78. True	86. True	94. False
71. True	79. True	87. True	95. False
72. False	80. True	88. False	96. True
73. True	81. True	89. False	97. False
74. False	82. True	90. False	98. False
75. True	83. True	91. False	99. False
76. True	84. False	92. False	100. True

Matching Type Questions

Part A

1.	H	6.	B
2.	G	7.	F
3.	E	8.	A
4.	D	9.	J
5.	C	10.	I

Part B

1.	F	6.	A
2.	G	7.	E
3.	C	8.	H
4.	D	9.	I
5.	A	10.	J

Part C

1.	D	6.	G
2.	C	7.	H
3.	A	8.	F
4.	B	9.	J
5.	E	10.	I

Part D

1.	H	6.	C
2.	J	7.	D
3.	B	8.	G
4.	I	9.	E
5.	A	10.	F

Part E

1.	B	6.	E
2.	A	7.	H
3.	D	8.	G
4.	C	9.	J
5.	F	10.	I

Part F

1.	J	6.	A
2.	I	7.	B
3.	H	8.	C
4.	G	9.	D
5.	F	10.	E

www.ingramcontent.com/pod-product-compliance
Ingram Content Group UK Ltd.
Pitfield, Milton Keynes, MK11 3LW, UK
UKHW021953270726
14060UKWH00002B/498

9 789351 246565